RAINBOW VEGAN COOKBOOK

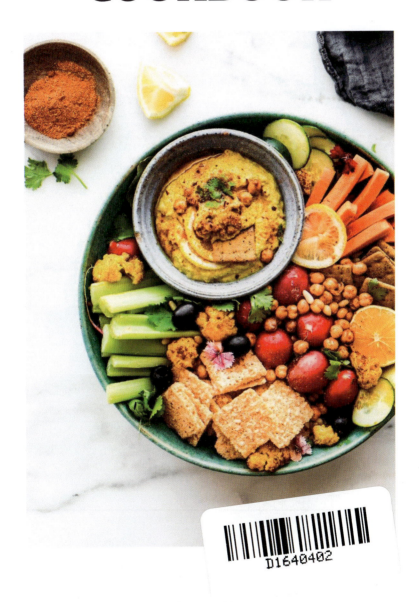

RAINBOW VEGAN RECIPE COOKBOOK:

Easy Plant Based Healthy Vegan Recipes for Everybody. Best 7 Days Vegan Diet (+ Simple Meal Plan for Vegans for Weight Loss, Detox, Cleanse and Healthy Life)

Anna Bright

Copyright ©[Anna Bright]

All rights reserved. No part of this guide may be reproduced in any form without permission in writing from the publisher except in the case of brief quotations embodied in critical articles or reviews.

Legal & Disclaimer

The information contained in this book and its contents is not designed to replace or take the place of any form of medical or professional advice; and is not meant to replace the need for independent medical, financial, legal, or other professional advice or services, as may be required. The content and information in this book have been provided for educational and entertainment purposes only.

The content and information contained in this book have been compiled from sources deemed reliable, and it is accurate to the best of the Author's knowledge, information, and belief. However, the Author cannot guarantee its accuracy and validity and cannot be held liable for any errors and/or omissions. Further, changes are periodically made to this book as and when needed. Where appropriate and/or necessary, you must consult a professional (including but not limited to your doctor, attorney, financial advisor or such other professional advisor) before using any of the suggested remedies, techniques, or information in this book.

Upon using the contents and information contained in this book, you agree to hold harmless the Author from and against any damages, costs, and expenses, including any legal fees potentially resulting from the application of any of the information provided by this book. This disclaimer applies to any of the loss, damages or injury caused by the use and application, whether directly or indirectly, of any advice or information presented, whether for breach of contract, tort, negligence, personal injury, criminal intent, or under any other cause of action.

You agree to accept all risks of using the information presented in this book.

You agree that, by continuing to read this book, where appropriate and/or necessary, you shall consult a professional (including but not limited to your doctor, attorney, or financial advisor or such other advisor as needed) before using any of the suggested remedies, techniques, or information in this book.

CONTENTS

INTRODUCTION 1

CHAPTER 1 THE BASICS OF THE VEGAN DIET 3

BENEFITS OF LIVING A VEGAN LIFESTYLE 4
HEALTH BENEFITS OF FOLLOWING A VEGAN DIET 4
INCREASED ENERGY 4
HEALTHIER SKIN 5
WEIGHT LOSS 5
IMPROVED HEART HEALTH 5
IMPROVED BRAIN HEALTH 6

CHAPTER 2 DIFFICULTIES AND CHALLENGES OF A VEGAN DIET & LIFESTYLE 7

PERMISSIBLE & NON- PERMISSIBLE ITEMS OF A VEGAN DIET 8
HOW TO ACHIEVE OPTIMAL NUTRITION IN THE VEGAN DIET 9
NEED FOR VEGAN SUPPLEMENTS 12
MISTAKES TO AVOID 12

CHAPTER 3 TIPS WHILE TRANSITIONING 13

CHAPTER 4 VEGAN RECIPES 16

10 VEGAN PORRIDGES 16
    Apple Pie Porridge 16
    Chocolate Strawberry Oatmeal 18
    Overnight Blueberry Oats 20
    Vegan Keto Porridge 22
    Pear & Walnut Oatmeal 24
    Overnight Golden Milk Oats 26
    Easy Vegan Oatmeal 28
    Vegan Quinoa Breakfast Porridge with Strawberries 30
    Healthy Oatmeal 32
    Overnight Coconut Latte Oats 34

10 VEGAN SALADS 36
    Kale & Sweet Potato Salad 36
    Buckwheat Noodle Salad 38
    Quinoa Cranberry Salad 40
    Cobb Salad 42
    Roasted Squash & Chickpea Salad 45
    Greens, Avocado & Strawberry Salad 47

Zucchini Ribbon & Lentil Salad	49
Roasted Beet & Spinach Salad	51
Broccoli Salad with Peanuts	53
Brussels Sprouts, Apple & Walnut Salad	55

10 Vegan Snacks 57

Almond & Nuts Granola Bar	57
Blueberry Quinoa Bran Muffins	59
Apple & Sweet Potato Hash	61
Pumpkin Biscuits	63
Chocolate Chunk Cookies	65
Kale Chips	67
Grilled Eggplant	69
Cheesy Chili Baked Potatoes	71
Tofu Meatballs	73
Apricot Almond Bars	75
Energy Balls	77
Baked Donuts	79
Celeriac Fries	81

10 Vegan Soups 83

Turmeric & Lentil Soup	83
Roasted Tomato Soup	85
Sweet Potato Soup	87
Broccoli Bisque	89
Black Bean Soup	91
Creamy Asparagus Soup	93
Arugula Artichoke Soup	95
Cauliflower Tomato Soup	97
Curried Corn Chowder	99
Carrot Soup	101

10 Vegan Main Meals 103

Vegan Banana Bread	103
Chickpea Omelet	105
Vegan Pancakes	107
Tofu Scramble	109
Chickpea Patties	111
Coconut Curry	113
Spinach-Parmesan Casserole	115
Spanakopita Mashed Potatoes	117
Tomato & Garlic Butter Beans	119
Spanish Spinach with Chickpeas	121

10 Vegan Desserts 123

Golden Milk Smoothie	123

Strawberry Chia Pudding... *125*
Sweet Potato Oatmeal *127*
Peanut Butter Oatmeal *129*
Carrot Cake Oatmeal... *131*
Savory Oatmeal *133*
Mint-Chip Coconut Milk Ice Cream *135*
Vegan Chocolate Ice Cream *137*
Orange Vegan Cake *139*
Vegan Strawberry Oatmeal Smoothie... *141*

10 VEGAN SAUSES **143**
Kale Walnut Pesto *143*
Vegan Ranch Dressing.. *145*
Vegan Nacho Cheese *147*
Ginger Cranberry Sauce... *149*
Vegan Green Chile Cilantro Sauce... *151*
Tomato sauce *153*
Chipotle Aioli.. *155*
Romesco Sauce.. *157*
Vegan Chocolate Sauce *159*
Miso–Ginger Sauce.. *161*

7-DAY VEGAN MEAL PLAN **163**

CONCLUSION... **164**

INTRODUCTION

The vegan diet is applauded by many because of the nutritional benefits that come with being on this diet. Many people view vegans as people who are extremely passionate about animals and the impact that the mass production of animals, especially cattle, has on the environment. The vegan lifestyle transcends animal rights issues and has a direct impact on individuals' overall health and well being. Most of the chronic diseases that many people struggle with are a result of being on a meat-oriented diet which usually leads to the consumption of lots of processed foods which add little nutrional value to the body and contribute to the dysfunction of bodily systems.

Dairy and meat products are known to contain high levels of saturated fats that contribute to conditions such as type 2 diabetes and heart-related diseases among others. Adopting a vegan lifestyle puts one on a path where they consume only plant-based foods that are not only nutritious but also contribute to overall good health. The vegan diet is high in fiber, and the filling nature of high fiber diets helps with weight loss issues since one is more likely to feel full most of the time. Therefore it means that a reduced intake of calories can be attained without feeling hungry.

The Rainbow Vegan Cookbook shares in detail what the vegan diet is all about, the benefits of adopting the vegan lifestyle and the health benefits that come with being on the diet. To succeed with this lifestyle, one needs a lot of information about what the diet entails, and how they can successfully prepare as they transition from a meat- and dairy-based diet to a plant-based one. The transition process may not be easy for someone who has been consuming dairy since infancy. However this book sheds light on how you can gradually transition to replacing the foods that might be your favorites before you decide on the vegan diet.

This book also offers delicious vegan recipes that you can prepare to help you succeed with the diet. In addition to reading this book, you also need facts on the subject from which you can draw vital information. One of the key things to focus on is ensuring that you meet the recommended nutritional requirements so that you don't end up being deficient in any valuable vitamins or nutrients. As shared in the book, you will get to learn about the common mistakes that people make, and how you can avoid them so as to succeed with the vegan lifestyle.

Whether you are on the vegan diet to lose weight, improve your level of mental clarity or reap the myriad benefits that come with being on the diet, you will get valuable information that will keep you on the path to success with the vegan diet.

Chapter 1

The Basics of the Vegan Diet

The vegan diet continues to soar in popularity with many people opting for the diet due to the various benefits it offers. When practiced right, the diet yields lots of benefits including weight loss and improved control of blood sugar. The vegan diet is a plant- based diet that excludes all forms of animal products including dairy, eggs and meat. Apart from the health benefits, many people adopt the vegan diet for ethical and environmental reasons.

Various studies have proven that the vegan diet has great health benefits if well planned, and those who have been on diets that are rich in dairy and meat can realize significant changes in the body by shifting to the vegan diet. One outstanding shift is a boost of energy which occurs when one eliminates the intake of processed foods and other elements of common diets. There are different types of vegan diets, the common ones being:

Whole-food vegan diet: This is a diet based on a wide range of whole plant foods such as whole grains, vegetables, legumes, and nuts and seeds.

Raw-food vegan diet: This vegan diet is based on raw fruits, seeds, vegetables, nuts and other plant foods that may be cooked at temperatures below 118^0F.

80/10/10: This is a raw food vegan diet that limits consumption of fat-rich plants such as avocados and nuts. Those on the diet rely on intake of raw fruits and soft greens. The diet is also referred to as "fruitarian" or low-fat, raw-food vegan diet.

There are other variations of vegan diets, however the common ones are the first two which are the raw-food and whole-food diets.

BENEFITS OF LIVING A VEGAN LIFESTYLE

People are constantly on the lookout for healthy eating lifestyles that they can adopt, and the vegan diet is the best option for many people because of the fantastic health benefits that those living the lifestyle experience. Apart from the health benefits, living a vegan lifestyle is also beneficial to the environment around us. The production of meat and animal products tends to place significant pressure on the environment due to use of water and crops required to ensure the animals are well fed, and to their waste

Living a vegan lifestyle is, therefore, not only beneficial to an individual but also has great benefits for the environment. The use of chemicals and antibiotics is common in processed meat production and hence tends to have a negative impact on overall health and well being. Adopting a vegan lifestyle, therefore, helps one to avoid conditions that might otherwise occur as a result of consuming processed meats.

HEALTH BENEFITS OF FOLLOWING A VEGAN DIET

The benefits that come with following a vegan diet impact both internal and external well-being The internal benefits include aspects such as improved cardiovascular health, reduced risks of type 2 diabetes and controlled blood pressure. There are, however, more obvious benefits that one experiences just after a few weeks of being on the diet. Here are some of the benefits:

INCREASED ENERGY

Adopting a vegan diet leads to increased energy levels. The consumption of heavily processed foods and sugars has the potential of leaving one feeling tired and sluggish after a short time. A switch to plant-based foods enhances energy levels, and one feels more energetic and focused most of the time.

HEALTHIER SKIN

Being on a vegan diet improves skin health as the vegan foods have nutrients that help to keep the skin healthy and glowing. Vitamin A-rich foods enhance skin health because it increases blood-flow to the skin surface which in turn reduces signs of aging and firms up the skin. Foods such as carrots, sweet potatoes and kale are great sources of vitamin A.

WEIGHT LOSS

Weight loss is another key benefit of a vegan diet. Plant-based diets are rich in fiber which makes them quite filling. It, therefore, means that one will feel full longer with less of a chance of craving snacks before meal times. Many people on typical western diets with processed foods and saturated fats tend to feel hungry often. Since their foods are not rich in fiber, it leads to unhealthy cravings and hinders weight loss. Adopting a vegan diet, therefore, translates into weight loss that can be sustained over time.

IMPROVED HEART HEALTH

Cardiovascular diseases are some of the chronic illnesses in the modern world. Being on a vegan diet can have a significant impact on the heart's health and the blood vessels. Eating vegetables and nutritious plant- based foods provides nutrients that the cardiovascular system needs to function well. Consumption of legumes and nuts also help with keeping the blood pressure at an optimal level. People on a vegan diet are likelier to experience fewer cases of stroke as one feels energized most of the time.

IMPROVED BRAIN HEALTH

Most people on a vegan diet tend to feel less anxious and have improved mental stability. Brain fogginess that frequently occurs when one is on a meat-based diet is not common with those on a vegan diet. That is because most of the vegan foods are rich in Vitamins D, B12 and A which are essential for proper functioning of the brain.

Chapter 2

Difficulties and Challenges of a Vegan Diet & Lifestyle

Even though a vegan diet provides a wide range of benefits, there are challenges that one can experience if the diet is not properly planned. A well-planned vegan diet should limit intake of processed foods and focus more on nutrient-rich foods. A poorly planned vegan diet may lead to certain nutrient deficiencies and a higher risk of having inadequate levels of vitamin B12, calcium, zinc, iodine, Vitamin D and the long-chain omega-3s. This can put the body at greater risks.

Lack of such nutrients may pose a great risk to children, and to breastfeeding and pregnant women since they have increased requirements for these nutrients. To minimize the chances of experiencing deficiency, there should be a limited intake of vegan processed foods with priority given to the nutrient-rich plant foods. One should commit to consuming nutrient-rich foods and also embracing cooking practices that enhance absorption of the nutrients. Some common challenges include struggling to give up favorite foods and adjusting to the taste of the available substitutes. Dairy products can be difficult to replace since the attributes of dairy foods come mostly from fats and proteins. Most people start consuming these foods right from infancy, so the taste is somehow deeply ingrained. There is also a distinct difference between milk-based and soy-based products. Lack of social support is another challenge that many people face when adopting the vegan lifestyle.

Vitamin B12 deficiency is a challenge that many people opting for a vegan diet contend with since its main source is meat. To address this challenge, fortified foods that are enriched with

Vitamin D, Calcium and Vitamin B12 should be consumed daily. Addition of iodized salt or seaweed can help with reaching the required iodine daily intake.

PERMISSIBLE & NON- PERMISSIBLE ITEMS OF A VEGAN DIET

To achieve all the benefits that come with being on a vegan diet, it's advisable that one has a good understanding of what the diet entails, and what needs to be done if success is to be realized.

Here are some of the foods that should be avoided:

- **Meat and poultry**: Includes lamb, pork, beef, chicken, turkey and all other meat products.
- **Fish and seafood**: All types of fish
- **Dairy**: All dairy products such as butter, cream, milk, yoghurt and cheese
- **Eggs**: All types of eggs
- **Bee products**
- **Animal-based ingredients**

Foods that should be consumed:

- Fruits and vegetables
- Fermented and sprouted plant foods
- Whole grains and cereals
- Algae
- Nutritional yeast
- Nuts and nut butters
- Seeds
- Calcium fortified plant milks and plant-milk yoghurts
- Legumes
- Tofu, tempeh and seitan

How to Achieve Optimal Nutrition in the Vegan Diet

Vegan diets are ideal for anyone regardless of age or stage of life. A healthy vegan diet is capable of meeting one's nutritional needs regardless of the stage one is in, whether pregnant, breastfeeding or even older adults.

To have a well-planned vegan diet that has the potential of meeting all of the nutritional needs, the following items should be taken into account:

Protein

Protein-rich foods are vital for overall health and help to keep the red blood cells and muscles healthy. Protein helps to support growth throughout one's life cycle. The sources of protein on a vegan diet include:

- Soy and soy products such as tofu, and soy fortified beverages.
- Meat alternatives such as veggie burgers and textured vegetable protein
- Dried beans such as black, white and kidney beans. Peas such as chickpeas, and black-eyed peas. Lentils such as green, red and brown lentils.
- Nuts and nut butters such as hazelnuts and almond butter. Seeds such as sunflower and sesame seeds.
- Peanuts and peanut butter.

Iron

Iron helps the blood carry oxygen to the different parts of the body. Those on a vegan diet require almost twice as much dietary iron as those on a non-vegan diet. This is because the iron extracted from the plant-based foods is not as well absorbed into the body as those from animal-based foods. For this nutritional requirement to be met, vegans need to choose foods on a daily basis that are rich in iron. The vegan sources of iron are absorbed better when one is also eating foods that are rich in vitamin C.

Foods that are rich in vitamin C include oranges, grapefruit and their juices, limes, kiwis, lemons, mangos, leafy vegetables like broccoli and more. The foods that are rich in iron include:

- Soy and soy products
- Dried beans
- Meat alternatives
- Fortified grain products
- Nuts and seeds
- Juices such as prune juice, and apricot juice
- Vegetables such as kale, spinach and potatoes
- Blackstrap molasses.

Vitamin B12

This nutrient is important for making red blood cells and helps the body use fats. Some of the good sources of vitamin B12 include:

- Nutritional yeast
- Fortified soy beverages and fortified non-dairy beverages
- Fortified meat alternatives.

Vitamin D

"Vitamin D" enables the body to absorb and also use calcium and phosphorus for development of strong healthy bones and teeth. Some of the good sources of vitamin D include:

- Fortified soy beverages and non-dairy beverages.
- Non-hydrogenated margarines
- Sunlight

Calcium

Calcium enables growth of healthy bones and overall health. It also enhances muscle contraction and heart beat. Good sources of calcium while on a vegan diet include:

- Soy yoghurt, fortified soy beverages and other non-diary beverages.
- Soy beans
- Almonds
- Blackstrap molasses
- Leafy vegetables, collard greens, turnip greens, bok choy and more
- Fortified orange juice, figs.

Zinc

Zinc is needed for growth and development of the body. It also helps in strengthening the immune system and healing wounds. Sources of zinc include:

- Soy and soy products
- Dried beans
- Nuts and peanuts
- Seeds
- Whole grains and fortified cereals

Omeg-3 Fats

Omega-3 fats are vital for brain, nerve and eye development. They also help with prevention of heart related diseases. Sources of omega-3 fats include:

- Oils such as flax seed, soybean and walnut
- Ground flax seed
- Soybeans, tofu and walnuts

NEED FOR VEGAN SUPPLEMENTS

There are some vegans that may find it a challenge to eat fortified foods or nutrient rich ones. Intake of supplements can be considered in such cases. Here are some of the supplements that can be considered;

- Vitamin B12
- Vitamin D
- Iron
- Calcium
- Iodine
- Zinc

Intake of supplements is only advisable where cases of deficiency have been identified. Too much intake of the supplements may cause complications if not well monitored.

MISTAKES TO AVOID

Here are some common mistakes that many people on a vegan diet often make;

- Assuming that all vegan products are automatically healthy.
- Failing to get enough vitamin B12
- Replacing meat products with cheese
- Consuming too few calories
- Failure to drink enough water
- Not eating enough of whole foods
- Consuming diets with low levels of calcium

To have a well planned vegan diet, you need to address all of the mistakes by ensuring the right nutrient-based foods are consumed and in the right proportions.

Chapter 3

Tips while transitioning

Before you start off with the process of transitioning to a vegan diet, you need to familiarize yourself well with the vegan diet. Having sufficient knowledge is vital as that will enable you to handle each process of the transition well. Here are some things you need to learn:

Benefits of adopting a vegan lifestyle: You need to learn about the benefits that come with being on a vegan diet including the costs and practices behind the production of animal-based products.

Optimal nourishment: Learn about how you can stay nourished with plant-based foods. Get to know the foods that you need to eat to stay nourished and which should be avoided.

Read ingredients lists: Your nourishment highly depends on the quality of foods that you eat. You should therefore have clear understanding of food compositions and the ingredients used in making foods.

Look for vegan products within your locality: To sustain the vegan lifestyle, you will need a local supply of vegan foods. You therefore need to be on the lookout for vegan products within your locality.

As you begin the transition process, you can consider engaging in the following;

- Begin familiarizing yourself with vegan foods by incorporating more of them in your diet. Incorporate more legumes, beans, nuts, whole grains, seeds and tofu into your diet. You should also familiarize yourself with the cooking methods, ingredients and storage.

- Begin collecting vegan recipes and experimenting with what appeals to you. Begin with meals that are easy to prepare and those you enjoy preparing.
- Switch milk to the non-dairy alternatives such as soy or almond. Experiment with the options available until you find what you prefer.

To start with the transition, you need to eliminate all the meat products in your diet including poultry and fish. Focus more on including plant based sources of protein. You may also continue to eat eggs and dairy products for a short time as you complete doing away with meat products. As you transition, try to avoid the common mistakes that many people make by resorting to plant-based foods that have been processed. You will not meet nutritional requirements if you focus on consuming processed plant-based foods.

Once you have successfully phased out meat products from your diet and you are comfortable, you can then focus on phasing out dairy products, eggs and honey. Choose one food group at a time until you successfully manage to phase it out, then proceed to the next.

To make the transition process comfortable, gradually phase out the animal and dairy products. You also need motivation and a positive mental attitude to keep progressing well. Focus on the ingredients and phase out ingredients derived from animal products. Once you have successfully managed to phase out all the unwanted food products, the next step is to practice the vegan lifestyle.

To succeed with the "veganism" lifestyle, have a list of the wide range of foods that you can choose from and a list of foods that you must consume daily to meet the recommended nutritional requirements. Information is vital, so look for support groups which have vital information that you can draw insight and support from as you start off with your vegan lifestyle.

Chapter 4

Vegan Recipes

10 Vegan Porridges

Apple Pie Porridge

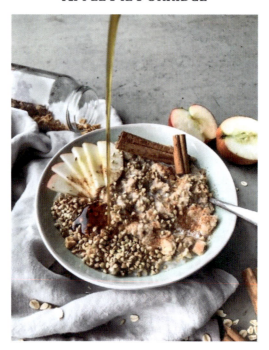

Preparation Time: 10 Minutes
Cooking Time: 10 Minutes
Servings: 1

Ingredients:

- Green Apple, organic, peeled & cored -1
- Almond Milk -1/2 cup

- Coconut Sugar -1/2 tablespoon
- Chia Seeds-2 tablespoons
- Cinnamon, ground-1/2 teaspoon
- Almond Butter -2 tablespoons
- Mixed Spices -1/2 teaspoon
- Pecans, for toppings

Method of Preparation:

1. In a high-speed blender add all the ingredients except pecans and blend for 4 minutes or until smooth and well mixed.
2. Put the mixture to a saucepan and heat over medium-low heat.
3. Remove from heat once warm.
4. Spoon the porridge into a bowl and garnish with chopped pecans.

Tip: You can also top it with apples or blueberries.

Nutritional Information per serving:

- Calories: 383 Kcal
- Carbohydrates: 36.2 g
- Fat: 28.5 g
- Proteins: 8.1 g

Chocolate Strawberry Oatmeal

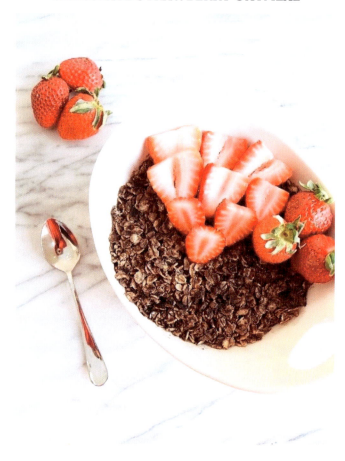

Preparation Time: 2 Minutes
Cooking Time: 10 Minutes
Servings: 1

Ingredients:

- Vegan Dark Chocolate, chopped -1 tablespoon
- Rolled Oats -1/3 cup
- Cocoa Powder-1 tablespoon
- Banana, mashed -1
- Strawberries, diced-1/4 cup
- Nut Milk -1/2 cup

Method of Preparation:

1. Place nut milk, oats, cocoa powder and mashed banana in saucepan and combine well.
2. Heat saucepan over medium heat and bring to a boil stirring frequently.
3. Lower hear and allow to simmer until all milk has been absorbed by the oats.
4. Cook for about 8 minutes while stirring.
5. Transfer to a serving bowl and top with diced strawberries.
6. Serve hot or warm.

Tip: You can top with chocolate chips if desired.

Nutritional Information per serving:

- Calories: 511 kcal
- Carbohydrates: 57 g
- Fat: 32 g
- Proteins: 8.9 g

OVERNIGHT BLUEBERRY OATS

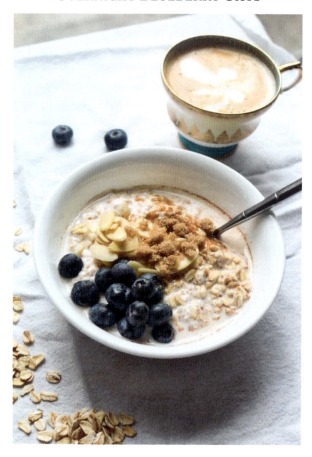

Preparation Time: 10 Minutes
Cooking Time: 5 Minutes
Servings: 2

Ingredients:

- Blueberries, fresh -1/2 cup
- Rolled Oats-1/2cup
- Chia Seeds-1 tablespoon
- Coconut Milk-1/2 cup
- Pinch of Salt
- Almond Milk -1/2cup

- Vanilla Extract -1 teaspoon
- Maple Syrup -2 tablespoons

Method of Preparation:

1. Place oats, maple syrup, chia seeds, salt, almond milk, and vanilla extract in a bowl and combine well.
2. Add the blueberries and fold in.
3. Transfer the mixture to mason jars and cover with lids
4. When ready to serve, top with shredded coconut or more blueberries.

Tip: You can also top with chia seeds.

Nutritional Information per serving:

- Calories: 377 Kcal
- Carbohydrates: 49 g
- Fat: 17 g
- Proteins: 8 g

Vegan Keto Porridge

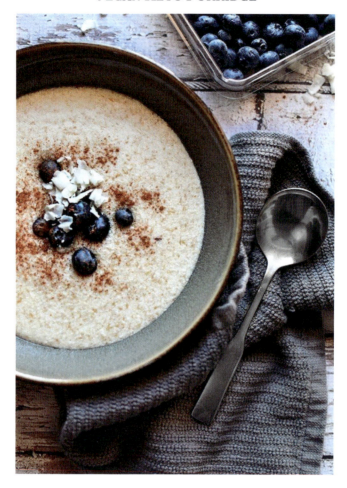

Cooking Time: 10 Minutes
Servings: 1

Ingredients:

- Almond Milk, unsweetened -1 1/2 cups
- Coconut Flour -2 tablespoons
- Erythritol, Powdered
- Golden Flax seed Meal-3 tablespoons
- Protein Powder-2 tablespoons

Method of Preparation:

1. In a bowl mix the flax seed, coconut flour, and protein powder until well combined.
2. Add the milk to the mixture and boil until thick.
3. Once cooked, add erythritol and toppings.

Nutritional Information per serving:

- Calories: 249 Kcal
- Carbohydrates: 3.78 g
- Fat: 13.07 g
- Proteins: 17 g

Pear & Walnut Oatmeal

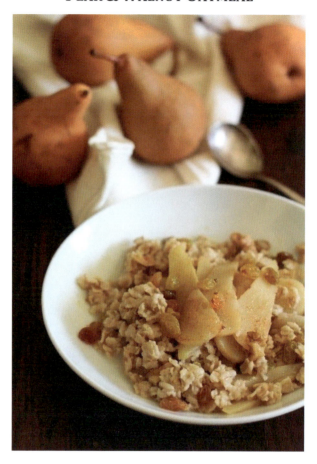

Preparation Time: 10 Minutes
Cooking Time: 5 Minutes
Servings: 1

Ingredients:

- Pear, organic, ripe & sliced -1
- Walnuts, chopped-2 teaspoons
- Rolled Oats -1/2 cup
- Cinnamon, ground-1/4 teaspoon
- Coconut Sugar-1 teaspoon

- Nut Milk -1 1/2 cups

For the sauce:

- Maple Syrup -1 tablespoon
- Coconut Oil -1 teaspoon
- Pinch of Salt
- Cocoa Powder-1 tablespoon

Method of Preparation:

1. Place oats in a saucepan and add the nut milk. Mix well.
2. Heat the saucepan over medium heat and cook for 4 minutes or until the mixture has thickened.
3. Then add the coconut sugar and cinnamon and stir well.
4. Meanwhile to make the sauce, mix all the ingredients listed in a small bowl until you get a fine smooth sauce.
5. Pour the cooked porridge into a serving bowl and top with sliced pear, walnut, and chocolate sauce.

Tip: Instead of pear, you can use banana.

Nutritional Information per serving:

- Calories: 396 Kcal
- Carbohydrates: 74 g
- Fat: 10 g
- Proteins: 9 g

Overnight Golden Milk Oats

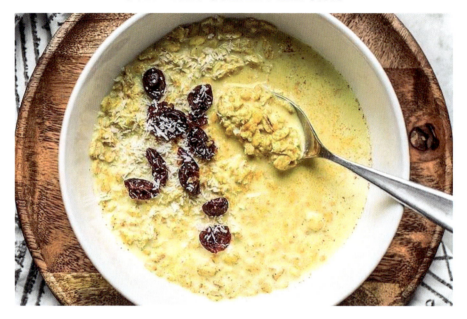

Preparation Time: 10 Minutes
Cooking Time: 15 Minutes
Servings: 2

Ingredients:

<u>For the golden milk:</u>

- Water, boiling -2 tablespoons
- Maple Syrup-1 tablespoon
- Cardamom, ground-1/4 teaspoon
- Nut Milk-2 cups
- Turmeric, ground-1 teaspoon
- Cinnamon, ground-1/4 teaspoon
- Ginger, ground-1/4 teaspoon

<u>For the Oats:</u>

- Hemp Hearts -2 tablespoons
- Rolled Oats -1 1/3 cups

- Golden Milk -1 1/2 cups
- Chia Seeds-2 tablespoons

Method of Preparation:

1. Mix maple syrup, cardamom, turmeric and ginger in a medium-sized bowl.
2. Combine them well and add the boiling water.
3. Pour in the nut milk and stir again.
4. Check for sweetness and add more syrup if needed.
5. Place oats, hemp hearts and chia seeds in a jar and shake well until combined.
6. Spoon the golden milk into the jar and shake again until everything comes together.
7. Place it in the refrigerator overnight.

Tip: Serve with fresh fruit as a topping.

Nutritional Information per serving:

- ➢ Calories: 447 Kcal
- ➢ Carbohydrates: 46.9 g
- ➢ Fat: 21.1 g
- ➢ Proteins: 20.2 g

Easy Vegan Oatmeal

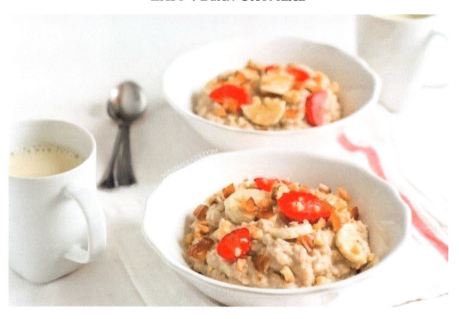

Preparation Time: 5 Minutes
Cooking Time: 10 Minutes
Servings: 1

Ingredients:
- Soy milk – 3/4 cup
- Oats – 1/4 cup
- Strawberry – 1, Medium Size
- Walnuts – 3, Whole
- Banana – 1, Medium
- Dates – 2, Whole
- Agave syrup – 1 teaspoon
- Cinnamon – 1/4 teaspoon

Method of Preparation:

1. Put milk into a saucepan and bring to a boil. Add oats and cook for 15 minutes over medium heat.

2. Place the mixture into a bowl and add the remaining ingredients. Stir well.
3. Serve and enjoy

Tip: Healthy and nutritious breakfast recipe

Nutritional Information per serving:

- ➢ Calories: 439 Kcal
- ➢ Carbohydrates: 73 g
- ➢ Fat: 13.1 g
- ➢ Proteins: 12.5 g

VEGAN QUINOA BREAKFAST PORRIDGE WITH STRAWBERRIES

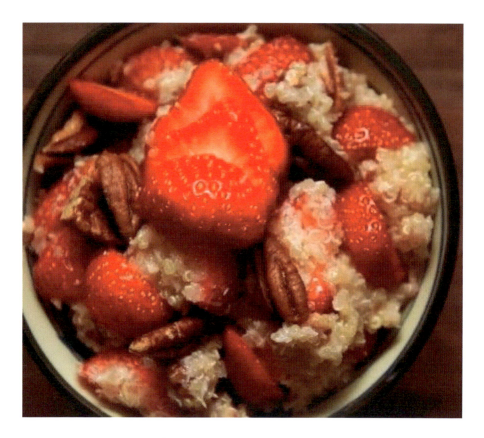

Preparation Time: 5 Minutes
Cooking Time: 15 Minutes
Servings: 2

Ingredients:

- Uncooked quinoa – 1 cup
- Almond or soy milk – 2 cups
- Agave nectar or brown sugar – 1 tablespoon
- Vanilla extract – ¼ teaspoon
- Dash cinnamon
- Strawberries – 1 cup
- Hazelnuts or pecans optional

Method of Preparation:

1. Put almond milk and quinoa in a saucepan, cover and cook over low heat, stirring occasionally, for about 10 minutes.
2. Add agave nectar or brown sugar, vanilla, and cinnamon and cook for 5 minutes or until quinoa is soft.
3. Stir in strawberries and healthy toppings, and serve.

Tip: A good reason for having leftover quinoa: you can easily prepare it with readily available ingredients.

Nutritional Information per serving:

- Calories: 450 Kcal
- Carbohydrates: 56 g
- Fat: 9.3 g
- Proteins: 7.8 g

HEALTHY OATMEAL

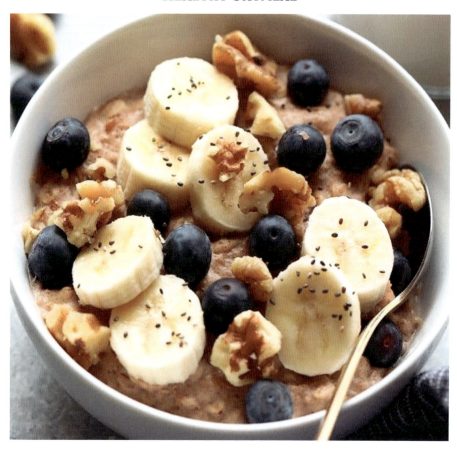

Preparation Time: 5 Minutes
Cooking Time: 5 Minutes
Servings: 2

Ingredients:

- Rolled oats – 1 cup
- Unsweetened almond milk – 1 medium
- Mashed banana – 1 medium
- Vanilla extract – ½ teaspoon
- Cinnamon – ½ teaspoon
- Pinch of salt

Method of Preparation:

1. In a saucepan, combine all ingredients and cook over medium heat.
2. When boiling, reduce heat to low and cook for 3 minutes or until it has thickened.
3. Once desired consistency is attained, remove from heat and serve immediately.
4. Top with banana slices

Tip: Add other flavors as desired to make it more delicious

Nutritional Information per serving:

- Calories: 238 Kcal
- Carbohydrates: 43 g
- Fat: 6 g
- Proteins: 7 g

Overnight Coconut Latte Oats

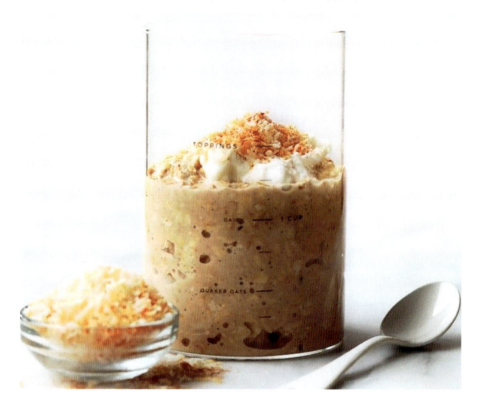

Preparation Time: 5 Minutes
Cooking Time: 0 Minutes
Servings: 2

Ingredients:

- Rolled oats – 1 cup
- Brewed coffee – ¼ cup
- Coconut milk – ¾ cup
- Maple syrup – 2 tablespoon
- Ground cinnamon – ½ teaspoon

Method of Preparation:

1. Place all the ingredients into a glass Tupperware bowl and mix.

2. Cover and refrigerate overnight.
3. Top with some coconut cream and shredded coconut including cinnamon
4. Enjoy

Tip: Very simple and easy to prepare recipe

Nutritional Information per serving:

- Calories: 26 1Kcal
- Carbohydrates: 43g
- Fat: 8 g
- Proteins: 5 g

10 Vegan Salads

Kale & Sweet Potato Salad

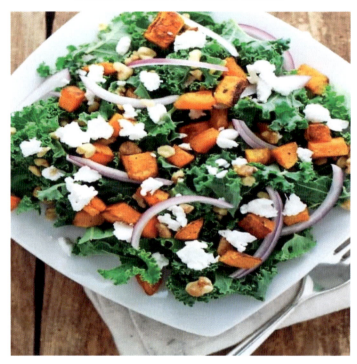

Preparation Time: 15 Minutes
Cooking Time: 40 Minutes
Servings: 4

Ingredients:

- Almonds, chopped-1/3 cup
- Salt, divided -3/4 teaspoon
- Sweet Potatoes, organic, medium & diced-2
- Cranberries, dried-1/3 cup
- Olive Oil, divided-3 tablespoons
- Red Onion, chopped-1/4 onion
- Juice of Lemon -1/2
- Avocado, organic, large & diced-1

- Black Pepper-1/4 teaspoon
- Bunch of Curly Kale, washed & chopped-1
- Garbanzo Beans -1 can (15 ounces)
- Quinoa, to serve

For the dressing:
- Salt-1/4 teaspoon
- Tahini Paste-1/2 cup
- Water -6 tablespoons
- Juice from Lemon-1

Method of Preparation:

1. Preheat the oven to 375°F.
2. Combine the diced sweet potatoes with 2 tablespoons of olive oil, pepper and ½ teaspoon of salt in a bowl.
3. Transfer the mixture to a sheet pan and bake for 40 minutes or until the sweet potatoes are tender. Flip the potatoes once.
4. Meanwhile, toss the kale with the remaining olive oil, salt and lemon juice in a bowl. Massage the kale with your hands for a minute to tenderize
5. Add all the dried nuts to it and toss again.
6. For the dressing, whisk all ingredients in a small mixing bowl until they become a smooth sauce.
7. Toss the kale with the sweet potato mixture in a large mixing bowl, drizzle the dressing over it and toss again.
8. Serve it with quinoa for a complete meal.

Tip: If the salad is stored properly in an air-tight container, it stays well in refrigerator for 5 days.

Nutritional Information per serving:

- Calories: 564 Kcal
- Carbohydrates: 42.7 g
- Fat: 41.3 g
- Proteins: 12.9 g

Buckwheat Noodle Salad

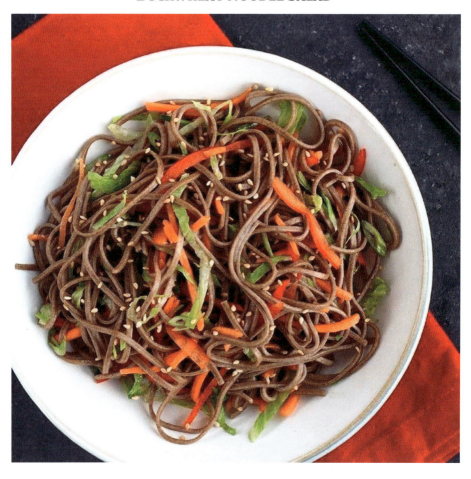

Preparation Time: 10 Minutes
Cooking Time: 15 Minutes
Servings: 2

Ingredients:

- Brown Rice Vinegar -1 tablespoon
- Buckwheat (soba) Noodles -2 cups
- Ginger, ground-1/4 teaspoon
- Boy Choy, small & chopped-1
- Sweet Corn -1 cup

- Sesame Oil -1 teaspoon
- Carrot, shaved -1/2 Cup
- Asparagus, shaved-2 cups
- Scallion, chopped-1/3 cup

Method of Preparation:

1. Cook the noodles according to the instructions given in the package.
2. Cook until al dente then drain.
3. Stir the rest of the ingredients into the cooked soba noodles and cook over medium heat, covered, for 5 minutes.
4. Transfer to a serving bowl and enjoy.

Tip: If possible, look for purple asparagus for better taste.

Nutritional Information per serving:

- Calories: 551 Kcal
- Carbohydrates: 89 g
- Fat: 7.6 g
- Proteins: 23.9 g

Quinoa Cranberry Salad

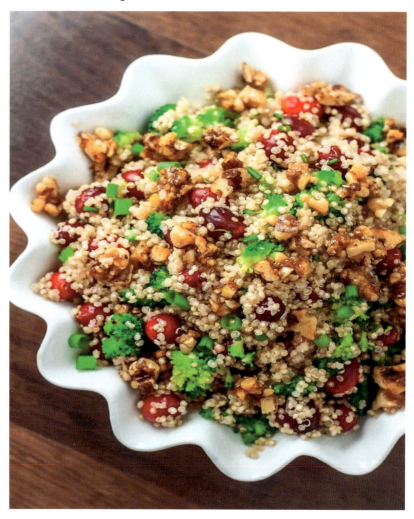

Preparation Time: 5 Minutes
Cooking Time: 10 Minutes
Servings: 6

Ingredients:

- Carrots, grated -1/2 cup
- Quinoa, washed & drained -1 cup
- Curry Powder-1 1/2 teaspoons

- Peanuts-2 Handful
- Vegetable Broth -1 1/2 cups
- Almonds, toasted & chopped-1/3cup
- Cranberries, dried-1/2 cup
- Red Onion, chopped-1/4 onion
- Cilantro, fresh & chopped-3 tablespoons
- Yellow Bell Pepper, diced-1/2 Cup
- Juice from Lemon -1
- Cumin -1/8 teaspoon
- Olive Oil, as desired
- Lime Wedges, as desired
- Salt-1/2 teaspoon
- Black Pepper, as desired

Method of Preparation:

1. Heat a pan of medium-size over medium heat and add the quinoa.
2. Toast it for few minutes or until dry.
3. Pour the broth into the pan and raise the heat to high.
4. Bring the mixture to a boil.
5. Once it starts boiling, reduce to low heat and allow it to simmer for 14 minutes or until the quinoa is fluffy and soft.
6. Mix the cooked quinoa with the rest of the ingredients until everything is well mixed.
7. Serve it chilled.

Tip: Pair it with grilled tofu for a complete meal.

Nutritional Information per serving:

- Calories: 199 Kcal
- Carbohydrates: 30 g
- Fat: 6 g
- Proteins: 6 g

Cobb Salad

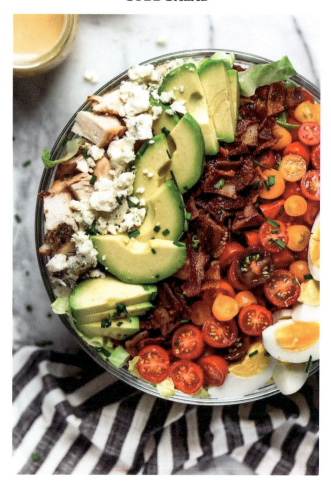

Preparation Time: 20 Minutes
Cooking Time: 15 Minutes
Servings: 4

Ingredients:

For the tofu:
- Tofu, extra firm, drained, pressed & cubed -1/2 lb
- Turmeric-1/4 teaspoon
- Salt-1/4 teaspoon
- Lemon Juice-2 teaspoons

- Garlic Powder-1/4 teaspoon
- Olive Oil -1 tablespoon
- Black Pepper-1/4 tablespoon

For the salad:
- Cherry Tomatoes, organic, large & halved -4
- Avocado, organic & quartered -1
- Chives, chopped-2 tablespoons
- Romaine Lettuce, chopped-1 head
- Chickpeas, cooked -1 cup
- Salt -1/2 teaspoon
- Green Bell Pepper, cubed-1/4 pepper
- Red Bell Pepper, cubed -1/4 pepper
- Yellow Bell Pepper, cubed -1/4 pepper

For the dressing:
- Maple Syrup -2 teaspoons
- Shallot, minced -2 tablespoons
- Black Pepper-1/4 teaspoon
- Water -1/4 cup
- Salt-1/2 teaspoon
- Olive Oil -1/4 cup
- Red Wine Vinegar -1/4 cup

Method of Preparation:

1. Begin by making the dressing: mix together all the ingredients listed in a small mixing bowl until smooth and set it aside.
2. Stir together salt, turmeric powder, garlic powder and pepper in a bowl.
3. Heat olive oil in a skillet of medium-size over medium heat.
4. Add the tofu and sauté for 10 minutes while flipping it once or twice.
5. Spoon in the lemon juice over the tofu and toss again.
6. Add turmeric powder over it and mix.
7. Place the lettuce, cooked tofu and all the remaining ingredients in a large mixing bowl.
8. Toss and drizzle with the dressing.

Tip: If you can get it, add coconut bacon for more taste and texture.

Nutritional Information per serving:

- Calories: 534 Kcal
- Carbohydrates: 36.3 g
- Fat: 43.9 g
- Proteins: 12.8 g

Roasted Squash & Chickpea Salad

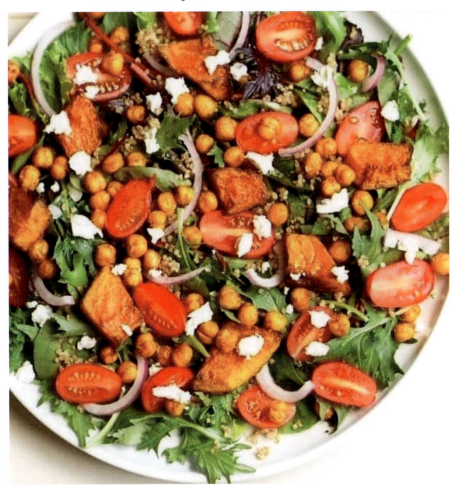

Preparation Time: 15 Minutes
Cooking Time: 20 Minutes
Servings: 6

Ingredients

- Butternut Squash, deseeded & sliced lengthwise-2 1/2 pounds
- Cumin, ground-1 teaspoon
- Red Onion, small & thinly sliced -1 onion

- Coriander Leaves, chopped-1/2 cup
- Olive Oil -1/3 cup
- Coriander, ground- 1 teaspoon
- Figs, chopped-6
- Zest & Juice of Lemon -1
- Chickpeas, washed & drained -3/4 Cup
- Salt -1 teaspoon

Method of Preparation:

1. Preheat the oven to 400°F.
2. Lightly grease a roasting pan with a tablespoon of olive oil.
3. Add the squash, coriander, 2 tablespoons of olive oil and cumin to a bowl.
4. Stir in salt and pepper and toss well.
5. Once mixed transfer it to a roasting pan and roast for 20 minutes or until the squash is tender. Set aside to cool.
6. Mix together chickpeas, onion, squash, coriander and figs in a large bowl.
7. Spoon in the remaining olive oil, lemon juice and zest, salt and pepper. Toss well and serve.

Tip: For a unique kick, you can add a pinch of turmeric powder.

Nutritional Information per serving:

- Calories: 258 Kcal
- Carbohydrates: 24 g
- Fat: 14 g
- Proteins: 6 g

Greens, Avocado & Strawberry Salad

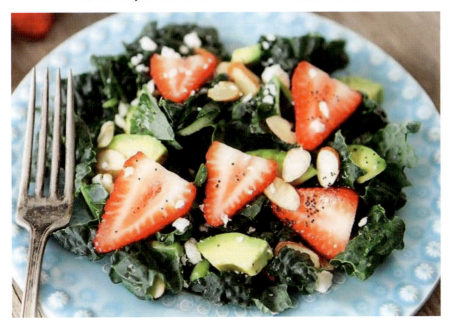

Preparation Time: 10 Minutes
Cooking Time: 10 Minutes
Servings: 2

Ingredients:

- Avocado, medium, ripe & diced -1
- Extra Virgin Olive Oil -1 1/2 teaspoons
- Balsamic Vinegar -1/3 cup
- Salad Greens, torn -1 cup
- Basil leaves -1/3 cup
- Strawberries, hulled & sliced -1 cup
- Black Pepper, to taste
- Sesame seeds, toasted, to serve, optional
- Cherry Tomatoes, halved -1 cup
- Himalayan Salt, to taste

Method of Preparation:

1. Start by simmering the vinegar in a small saucepan over medium heat.
2. Once it starts to simmer, lower the heat and allow it to simmer for another 8 to 10 minutes or until the vinegar has thickened and reduced by half. Set it aside.
3. In the meantime, toss strawberries, salad leaves, basil, avocado and tomatoes in a large mixing bowl.
4. Spoon in the olive oil and toss again gently.
5. Check for seasoning and add pepper and salt to taste.
6. Finally, drizzle the balsamic reduction over it and toss so that everything is well combined.

Tip: Garnish with toasted sesame seeds or chopped pecans if desired.

Nutritional Information per serving:

- Calories: 230 Kcal
- Carbohydrates: 28 g
- Fat: 15 g
- Proteins: 4 g

ZUCCHINI RIBBON & LENTIL SALAD

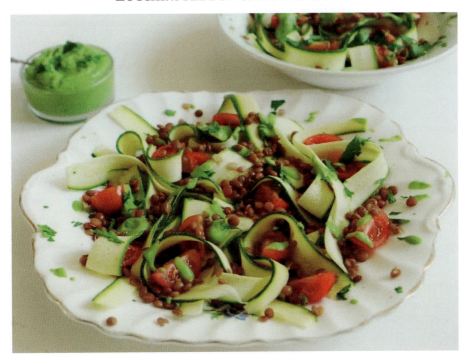

Preparation Time: 10 Minutes
Cooking Time: 10 Minutes
Servings: 1

Ingredients:

- Brown Lentils, cooked -1/2 cup
- Cherry Tomatoes, quartered -10
- Zucchini, sliced into ribbons with a vegetable peeler, ends discarded -2

For the dressing:
- Avocado, ripe & small-1
- Water -1/4 cup
- Parsley, fresh -1/2 cup
- Capers-15
- Garlic Powder-1/2 teaspoon
- Juice of Lemon -1/2 tablespoon

- Extra Virgin Olive Oil -1 tablespoon

Method of Preparation:

1. Cook the lentils in a saucepan of water for half an hour.
2. Once cooked, drain the lentils.
3. Place the zucchini ribbons and tomatoes in a serving dish.
4. Make the dressing like that: place all the ingredients in a blender and blend on high speed for 2 to 3 minutes or until the dressing is smooth.
5. Check for seasoning in the dressing and correct if needed.
6. Finally, spoon in the cooked lentils and pour the dressing over the veggies. Toss once gently.

Tip: You can use any lentils of your choice.

Nutritional Information per serving:

- Calories: 432 Kcal
- Carbohydrates: 44.2 g
- Fat: 28.7 g
- Proteins: 12 g

Roasted Beet & Spinach Salad

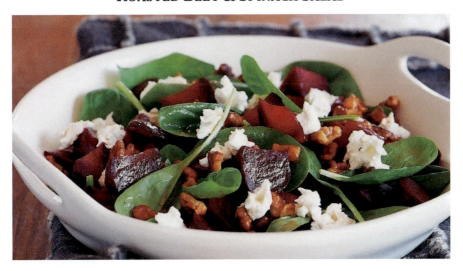

Preparation Time: 15 Minutes
Cooking Time: 30 Minutes
Servings: 6

Ingredients:

- Beets, small -10
- Extra Virgin Olive Oil -6 tablespoons
- Parsley, fresh -1/2 cup
- Agave Syrup -2/3 cup
- Garlic cloves, minced -3
- Red Wine Vinegar- 6 tablespoons
- Pumpkin Seeds, roasted -1/4 pound
- Green Beans, cooked -1/2 pound
- Sea Salt, as needed
- Baby Spinach -1/4 pound

Method of Preparation:

1) Preheat the oven to 400°F.
2) Wrap the beets in foil and cook them in the oven for an hour or until they become soft.
3) Once cooked, slice them into wedges.

4) Mix together the oil, agave syrup, garlic, and vinegar in a small mixing bowl.
5) Whisk the dressing well and check for seasoning. Correct if needed.
6) Finally, add the pumpkin seeds, green beans, beets, parsley and spinach to it.
7) Serve immediately.

Tip: Instead of red wine vinegar, you can also use sherry vinegar.

Nutritional Information per serving:

- Calories: 431 Kcal
- Carbohydrates: 53 g
- Fat: 23.1 g
- Proteins: 8.9 g

Broccoli Salad with Peanuts

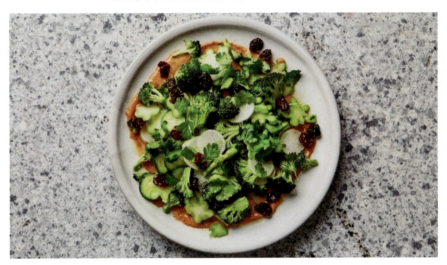

Preparation Time: 15 Minutes
Cooking Time: 15 Minutes
Servings: 4

Ingredients:

- Broccoli head, large & chopped into florets -1
- Peanuts -1/2 cup
- Edamame, shelled, cooked-1 cup
- Peanut Sauce (see below)
- Small Carrot, diced-1/2
- Green Onions, thinly sliced -1/2 cup
- Sesame Seeds, to garnish

For the peanut sauce:
- Rice Vinegar-1 tablespoon
- Toasted Sesame Oil -1/8 teaspoon
- Hot Water-2 tablespoons
- Peanut Butter-1/4 cup
- Agave Nectar-1 tablespoon
- Tamari -1 tablespoon

Method of Preparation:

1. Boil a pot of water over medium-high heat.
2. Once is starts boiling, add the broccoli florets and boil them for 25 to 30 seconds.
3. Strain the florets and place them in a bowl of ice water. Drain.
4. Place the drained florets in a bowl and add all the remaining ingredients. Toss to combine the ingredients well.
5. To make the sauce: Whisk all the ingredients in a small mixing bowl until you get a smooth sauce. If your peanut sauce seems too thick, add more hot water as needed. Pour the sauce over the florets mix. Toss to combine well.

Tip: You can even add slivered almonds to it for crunchier texture.

Nutritional Information per serving:

- Calories: 220 kcal
- Carbohydrates: 13 g
- Fat: 14.8 g
- Proteins: 12.4 g

BRUSSELS SPROUTS, APPLE & WALNUT SALAD

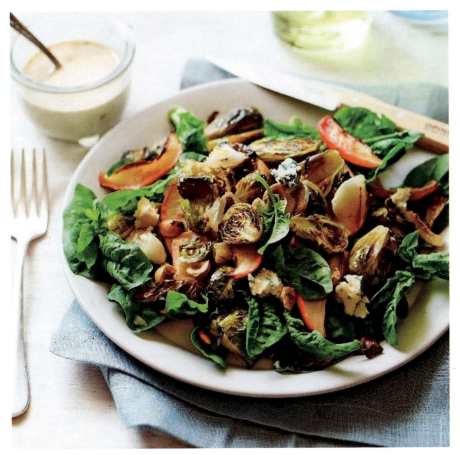

Preparation Time: 15 Minutes
Cooking Time: 10 Minutes
Servings: 6

Ingredients:

- Red Onion, medium & shredded-1
- Brussels Sprouts, ends trimmed & shredded-1 lb
- Granny Smith Apple, medium & chopped-1
- Cranberries, dried -1/4cup
- Walnuts, chopped-1/4 cup

For the vinaigrette:

- Maple Syrup-2 tablespoons
- Extra Virgin Olive Oil -1/2 cup
- Dijon Mustard -1 tablespoon
- Garlic clove, finely minced-1
- Salt-1/2 teaspoon
- Red Wine Vinegar-3 tablespoons
- Black Pepper, to taste

Method of Preparation:

1. Combine red onion, Brussels sprouts, cranberries and apple together in a large bowl.
2. Toast the walnuts in a medium-sized skillet over medium heat for about 2 to 3 minutes or until lightly browned.
3. Add the toasted walnuts to the bowl and toss again.
4. Make the dressing: Place all the ingredients listed in a jar and close with the lid.
5. Shake the jar well until everything is well combined.
6. Finally drizzle the dressing over the salad and toss again.

Tip: Better when chilled in the refrigerator for ½ hour.

Nutritional Information per serving:

- Calories: 354 Kcal
- Carbohydrates: 20.6 g
- Fat: 29.6 g
- Proteins: 8 g

10 Vegan Snacks

Almond & Nuts Granola Bar

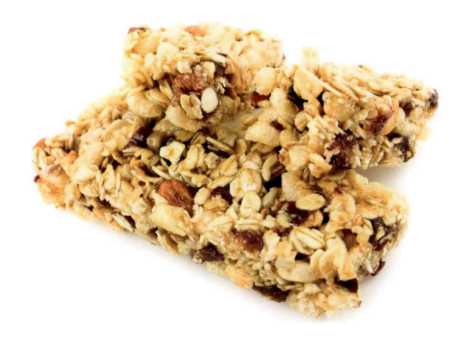

Preparation Time: 10 Minutes
Cooking Time: 35 Minutes
Servings: 8 Bars

Ingredients:

- Almond Butter-2 tablespoons
- Cinnamon -2 teaspoons
- Raisins-1 cup
- Date Syrup -5 tablespoons
- Bananas, organic,,ripe-3
- Sunflower Seeds-1/4 cup
- Oats -1 cup
- Pumpkin Seeds-1/2 cup
- Almonds-2/3 cup

- Flaxseeds-1/2 cup
- Puffed Brown Rice -1 cup

Method of Preparation

1. Preheated the oven to 375°F.
2. In a mixing bowl add pumpkin seeds, almonds, flax seeds, raisins and puffed rice and combine well.
3. In a food processor, add bananas, almond butter, and dates and blend the mixture for a minute or until well blended.
4. Spoon the mixture over the dry ingredients and combine well so that everything is sticky and well incorporated.
5. Transfer the mixture to a baking sheetwith parchment paper and spread it out.
6. Bake the mixture in the heated oven for 25 minutes, remove the baking sheet and cut the mixture into 8 bars with a knife.
7. Return them to the oven and bake until well browned.
8. Remove from oven and let them cool. You can store the bars in an air-tight container and serve when desired.

Tip: You could use maple syrup instead of date syrup.

Nutritional Information per serving:

- Calories: 339 Kcal
- Carbohydrates: 50 g
- Fat: 14.4 g
- Proteins: 10 g

Blueberry Quinoa Bran Muffins

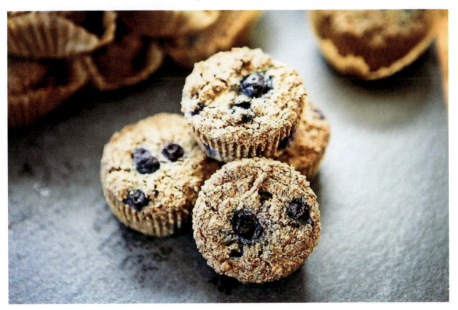

Preparation Time: 10 Minutes
Cooking Time: 40 Minutes
Servings: 12 Muffins

Ingredients:

- Blueberries, organic-1 cup
- Salt -1/2 teaspoon
- Quinoa Flour -1 cup
- Baking Soda -1 teaspoon
- Wheat Bran -1 cup
- Cinnamon -1 1/2 teaspoons
- Baking Powder-2 teaspoons
- Banana, ripe & mashed -1
- Vanilla Extract -1 teaspoon
- Coconut Milk -3/4 cup
- Molasses-1 tablespoon
- Apple Juice-1/2 cup
- Flax Seed Meal -1 tablespoon

Method of Preparation:

1. Preheat the oven to 350°F.
2. In a mixing bowl, add all of the dry ingredients except the blueberries and mix them well.
3. In another bowl, mix together the wet ingredients and blend until well combined.
4. Combine all of the ingredients together. Whisk them well until well combined.
5. Add the blueberries and gently fold in.
6. Grease a muffin pan lightly and pour the batter into the pan.
7. Bake the mixture for 20 minutes or until the muffins are well browned and a toothpick inserted in the centre comes out clean.
8. Remove them from the oven when ready and allow to cool slightly before serving.

Tip: Instead of coconut milk, you can choose any vegan milk.

Nutrient Information per serving:

- Calories: 82 Kcal
- Carbohydrates: 12.5 g
- Fat: 4.2 g
- Proteins: 1.7 g

APPLE & SWEET POTATO HASH

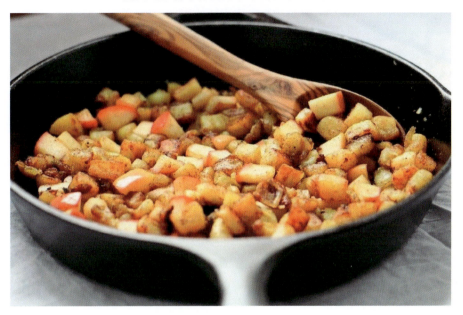

Preparation Time: 5 Minutes
Cooking Time: 10 Minutes
Servings: 4

Ingredients:

- Sage, chopped-1 tablespoon
- Sweet Potatoes, organic, large & cubed -2
- Salt-1/2 teaspoon
- Fuji Apple, organic, small & chopped-2
- Garlic Powder-1/2 teaspoon
- Coconut Oil -1/2 tablespoon
- Pinch of Black Pepper

Method of Preparation:

1. In a microwave-safe bowl, add cubed sweet potatoes and microwave for about 8 minutes on medium setting.

2. Place your skillet over medium heat and add coconut oil. Once the oil becomes hot, stir in the apples and sweet potatoes into the skillet.
3. Sauté the mixture for few minutes then add the sage.
4. Season it with salt and pepper and continue cooking for 8 minutes or until the apples and sweet potatoes are well cooked.
5. Transfer the sautéed sweet potatoes and apples to a serving bowl once ready and enjoy while hot.

Tip: Pair it with hemp hearts for a complete meal.

Nutritional Information per serving:

- ➢ Calories: 97 Kcal
- ➢ Carbohydrates: 19 g
- ➢ Fat: 1 g
- ➢ Proteins: 1 g

Pumpkin Biscuits

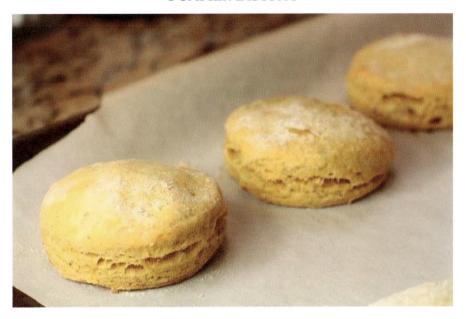

Preparation Time: 10 Minutes
Cooking Time: 15 Minutes
Servings: 14 Biscuits

Ingredients:

- Lime Juice-1 tablespoon
- Whole Wheat Flour -2 cups
- Raisins -1/4 cup
- Baking Powder-1 1/2 teaspoon
- Soy Milk, plain- 1/2 cup
- Baking Soda-1/2 teaspoon
- Nutmeg -1/2 teaspoon
- Pumpkin, puréed-1/2 cup
- Cinnamon, ground -1 1/4 teaspoons
- Cloves, ground -1/8 teaspoon
- Salt -1/2 teaspoon

Method of Preparation:

1. Heat the oven to 425°F.
2. In a bowl of large size mix together all of the dry ingredients and mix until well combined.
3. Add pumpkin to the mixture and mix until the mixture becomes well blended and crumbly.
4. Add to this the lemon juice and soy milk and mix well again until the dough becomes soft.
5. Prepare a floured surface. Add the dough and roll it to a thickness of about ¾ inch.
6. Once rolled, use a biscuit cutter to cut dough by pressing it straight down until you get to the surface.
7. Arrange the cut dough pieces on a baking sheet lined with parchment paper and bake them for about 10 minutes or until cooked.

Tip: To increase the sweetness, you can use stevia if desired.

Nutritional Information per serving:

- ➢ Calories: 75 Kcal
- ➢ Carbohydrates: 16 g
- ➢ Fat: 6 g
- ➢ Proteins: 3 g

Chocolate Chunk Cookies

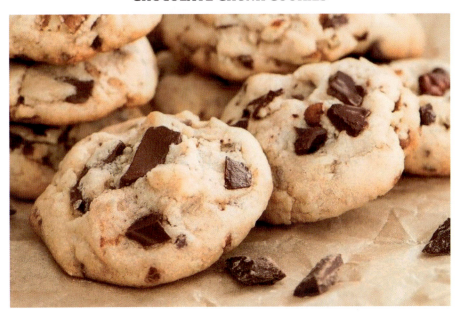

Preparation Time: 20 Minutes
Cooking Time: 10 Minutes
Servings: 13 Cookies

Ingredients:

- Vanilla Extract-1/2 teaspoon
- Maple Syrup -1/4 cup +3 tablespoons
- Almond Butter-1/2 cup
- Coconut Oil -3 tablespoons
- Baking Soda-1/2 teaspoon
- Rolled Oats-1/2 cup
- Almond Flour -1/4 cup
- Salt-1/2 teaspoon
- Oat Flour-1/4 cup + 3 tablespoons
- Arrowroot Flour-1/4 cup
- Chocolate Bar, non-diary, chopped -5 1/2 ounces

Method of Preparation:

1. Preheat the oven to 350°F.
2. In a large bowl mix together vanilla extract, maple syrup, almond butter and oil until well blended.
3. In another bowl add all the dry ingredients then combine and mix well.
4. Mix the dry ingredients and the wet ones together and blend until well combined. Add 3 tablespoons of chocolate into the mixture and stir until well mixed.
5. Line a baking sheet with parchment paper and using a scoop, place scoops of batter unto the parchment keeping some ample space between them. .
6. While you scoop the cookie dough press the remaining chocolate pieces over the tops of the cookies unevenly.
7. Bake in the preheated oven for about 8 minutes or until the cookies flatten out.
8. Remove from the oven. Aallow to rest for several minutes. You can serve at once or you can cool and keep in an airtight container.

Tip: If you want a crisper cookie, you can bake them for 12 minutes.

Nutritional Information per serving:

- Calories: 230 Kcal
- Carbohydrates: 22 g
- Fat: 15 g
- Proteins: 5 g

Kale Chips

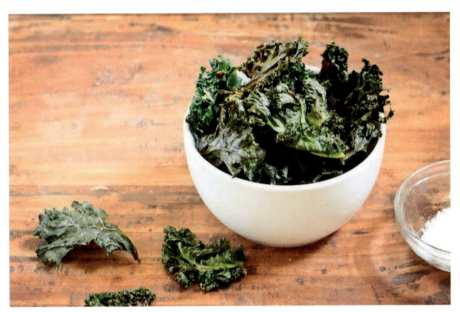

Preparation Time: 10 Minutes
Cooking Time: 25 Minutes
Servings: 1

Ingredients:

- Onion Powder -1/2 tablespoon
- Kale Leaves-1/2 bunch
- Himalayan Salt -1/4 teaspoon
- Extra Virgin Olive Oil -1/2 tablespoon
- Smoked Paprika-1/2 teaspoon
- Nutritional Yeast -1 1/2 tablespoons
- Chili Powder-3/4 teaspoon
- Garlic Powder-1 teaspoon

Method of Preparation:

1. Preheat the oven to 300°F.
2. Tear the kale leaves from the stems and wash the leaves carefully. Let them dry.

3. Place kale leaves in a bowl and add the oil over them.
4. Use your hands to coat the leaves well with olive oil. Sprinkle with the seasonings and toss to coat well.
5. Place the kale leaves onto a baking sheet that's lined with parchment paper and bake them for 9 minutes, then turn them over and bake for another 15 minutes to get a crispy texture.
6. Remove the sheet from the oven and allow the kale leaves to cool for a few minutes before serving.

Tip: For a bit of a kick, you can try adding a pinch of cayenne pepper.

Nutritional Information per serving:

- Calories: 78 Kcal
- Carbohydrates: 8 g
- Fat: 4.2 g
- Proteins: 4.6 g

Grilled Eggplant

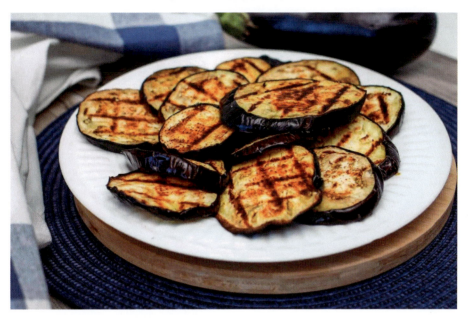

Preparation Time: 10 Minutes
Cooking Time: 10 Minutes
Servings: 4

Ingredients:

- Garlic Powder-1/2 teaspoon
- Eggplant, large & sliced into rounds-1
- Salt-1/2 teaspoon
- Cumin, ground-2 teaspoons

- Tamari-4 tablespoons
- Avocado Oil-2 tablespoons
- Coriander, ground-2 teaspoons

Method of Preparation:

1. Combine avocado oil and half of the tamari in a small bowl.

2. Apply the oil mixture over the sliced egg plant rounds and set aside.
3. Combine all of the remaining ingredients in a bowl and stir to incorporate well.
4. Add the spice mix to the eggplant rounds and coat them well.
5. Heat a grill to medium-high heat and place the eggplant rounds once the grill is hot. Cook them for 4 minutes per side or until the right texture is obtained.

Tip: For a spicy kick, you can add ½ teaspoon of Cayenne pepper.

Nutritional Information per serving:

- Calories: 94 Kcal
- Carbohydrate: 14 g
- Fat: 4 g
- Proteins: 2 g

Cheesy Chili Baked Potatoes

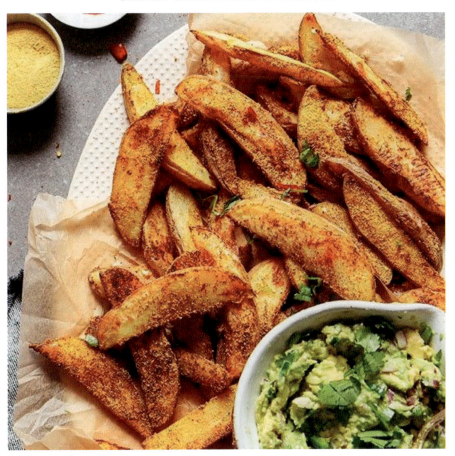

Preparation Time: 5 Minutes
Cooking Time: 35 Minutes
Servings: 6

Ingredients:

- Nutritional Yeas -3 tablespoons
- White Potatoes, sliced into wedges-2 1/2 pounds
- Sea Salt-1/2 teaspoon
- Chili Powder-1 teaspoon
- Dash of Cayenne Pepper
- Garlic Powder-1/2 teaspoon

- Water, as needed

Method of Preparation:

1. Preheat the oven to 425°F.
2. Place the potato wedges in a steamer over a pot of boiling water.
3. Cover and cook for 4 to 5 minutes or until the potatoes are slightly tender.
4. Transfer the potatoes to a large bowl and sprinkle them with the chili powder, garlic powder, nutritional yeast, cayenne pepper and salt.
5. Toss well.
6. Place the potatoes in a single layer on a baking sheet with ample space in between.
7. Bake them for 13 to 15 minutes. Remove the sheet from the oven and flip the potatoes once.
8. Finally, raise the heat to 450°F and bake for additional 10 to 12 minutes or until the potatoes are crisp and golden brown.

Tip: You can serve them along with guacamole and garnish with cilantro leaves if desired.

Nutritional Information per serving:

- Calories: 64 kcal
- Carbohydrates: 13.3 g
- Fat: 2.5 g
- Proteins: 2.9 g

Tofu Meatballs

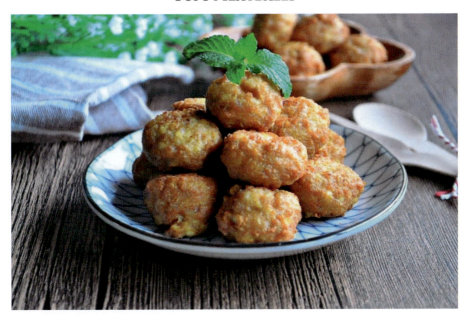

Preparation Time: 15 Minutes
Cooking Time: 35 Minutes
Servings: 6

Ingredients:

- Parsley, fresh -1/4 cup
- Bulgur Wheat, dry-3/4 cup
- Red Wine Vinegar-1 tablespoon
- Flax Meal, grounded-2 teaspoons
- Tofu, extra-firm -15 ounces
- Thyme, dried-2 teaspoons
- Nutritional Yeast-3 tablespoons
- Oregano, dried-1 tablespoon
- Black Pepper-1/4 teaspoon
- Sea Salt -1/4 teaspoon

Method of Preparation:

1. Place bulgur in a pot of water and heat it over medium-high heat.
2. Once the water starts boiling, reduce the heat to low.
3. Allow it to simmer for about 14 minutes with the pot covered.
4. Remove it from the heat once all the water has been absorbed and allow it to cool for several minutes.
5. Fluff it with a fork. Sset it aside for another 10 to 15 minutes.
6. Preheat the oven to 375°F.
7. Drain the tofu and place it in a food processor along with all the remaining ingredients, excluding parsley and flax meal. Process it until it becomes a smooth mixture.
8. Add the parsley and blend it again.
9. Finally, combine the tofu mixture with the cooked bulgur in a large mixing bowl, add the flax meal and mix by using your hands.
10. Make 30 to 40 balls out of this mixture and place them on a parchment lined baking sheet.
11. Bake them for 35 to 40 minutes or until crisp and browned.

Tip: If you wish, you could make it a big meal if you pair it with pasta.

Nutritional Information per serving:

- Calories: 135 Kcal
- Carbohydrates: 17.9 g
- Fat: 3.9 g
- Proteins: 10.6 g

APRICOT ALMOND BARS

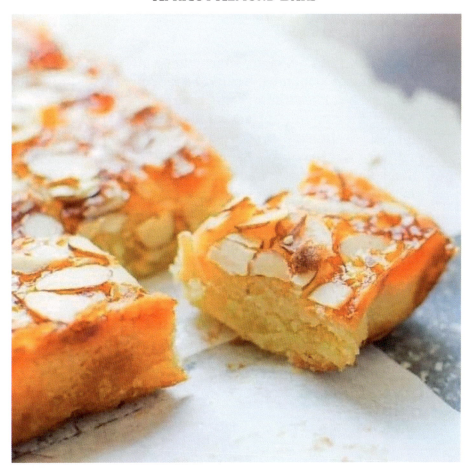

Preparation Time: 10 Minutes
Cooking Time: 20 Minutes
Servings: 12 Bars

Ingredients:

- Apricots, dried -8
- Almond Butter -1 tablespoon
- Almonds -1 1/2 cups
- Medjool Dates, pitted -10
- Salt -1/4 teaspoon
- Shredded Coconut, dried & unsweetened -2 tablespoons

- Vanilla Bean, split & seeds scraped out-1

Method of Preparation:

1. To make these delicious snack bars, you need to process the apricots, salt and almonds in a food processor until the mixture becomes a coarse meal.
2. Stir in the almond butter, vanilla bean chopped, coconut and dates into the processor and process it again for a minute or until you get a sticky mixture.
3. Transfer the mixture to a greased parchment paper-lined baking sheet and spread it evenly across the sheet.
4. Place the baking sheet in the refrigerator for an hour or until it is set.
5. Finally, slice it into bars.

Tip: If you want to keep it for few days, you could cover it with wax paper.

Nutritional Information per serving:

- Calories: 193 Kcal
- Carbohydrates: 29.9 g
- Fat: 7.3 g
- Proteins: 3.8 g

Energy Balls

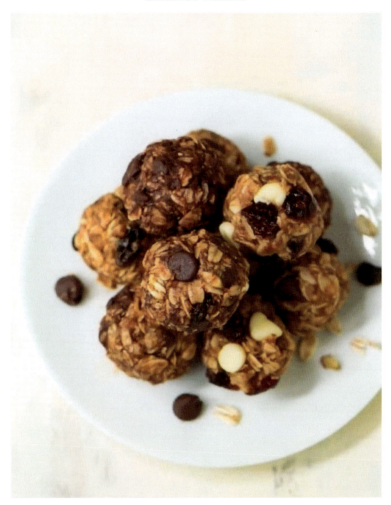

Preparation Time: 10 Minutes
Cooking Time: 15 Minutes
Servings: 12

Ingredients:

- Flax seeds-1 tablespoon
- Almonds -1/2 cup
- Tequila-2 tablespoons

- Walnuts-1/4 cup
- Zest of Lime-1
- Coconut Flakes-1/4 cup
- Lime Juice-2 teaspoons
- Coconut Shreds, dry-1/2 cup
- Mint Leaves-1/4 cup
- Chia Seeds-1 tablespoon
- Medjool Dates-9
- Sesame Seeds-1 tablespoon
- Salt -1/4 teaspoon

Method of Preparation:

1. Place the walnuts, flax seeds, almond and oats in a food processor and process until it becomes a coarse meal.
2. Add the dates, chia seeds, coconut, sesame seeds, salt and mint leaves and process them again or until you get a crumbly mixture.
3. Spoon in the tequila, lime juice and zest and blend for a minute or until you get a doughy mixture.
4. Transfer the dough to a bowl. If it seems too sticky, add oat flour.
5. Check for sweetness and add more sugar if needed.
6. Make balls out of this mixture and serve.

Tip: You can coat the balls with sesame seeds, if you desire more crunchiness.

Nutritional Information per serving:

- Calories: 145 Kcal
- Carbohydrates: 18 g
- Fat: 7 g
- Proteins: 2 g

BAKED DONUTS

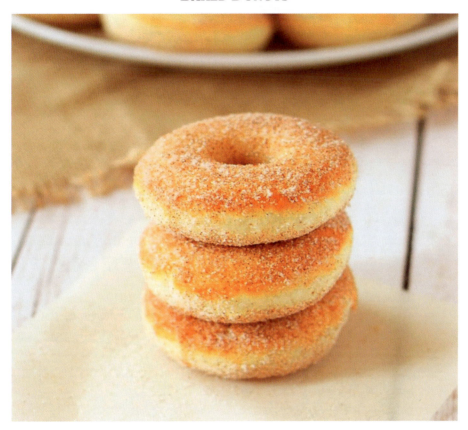

Preparation Time: 10 Minutes
Cooking Time: 10 Minutes
Servings: 12 Donuts

Ingredients:

- Apple Cider-3/4 cup
- All Purpose Flour -2 cups
- Coconut Oil, melted -1/2 cup
- Baking Powder-1 tablespoon
- Vanilla Extract -1 teaspoon
- Cinnamon -1/2 teaspoon
- Cashew Yoghurt -1/3 cup

- Nutmeg, grated freshly -1/4 teaspoon
- Coconut Sugar -1/3 cup
- Cardamom -1/4 teaspoon
- Cinnamon -1/2 teaspoon

For the topping:

- Cinnamon -1 tablespoon
- Sugar, granulated -1/2 cup
- Coconut Oil, melted -1/4 cup

Method of Preparation:

1. Preheat the oven to 350°F.
2. Take a large mixing bowl and stir in all the dry ingredients first and then the wet ingredients, excluding coconut oil, until everything is well incorporated.
3. Spoon in the coconut oil and mix again gently.
4. Pour the batter into a greased donut pan and bake for 13 minutes or until a toothpick inserted in the middle portion comes out clean.
5. Allow the donuts to cool in the pan for 10 minutes and then for another 10 minutes on a cooling rack.
6. In the meantime make the topping: mix together the cinnamon and sugar.
7. Finally, apply coconut oil over the dough nuts and immerse it in the cinnamon sugar.
8. Serve and enjoy.

Tip: Instead of cashew yoghurt, you can use coconut yoghurt.

Nutritional Information per serving:

- Calories: 241 Kcal
- Carbohydrates: 33 g
- Fat: 16.4 g
- Proteins: 2.4 g

CELERIAC FRIES

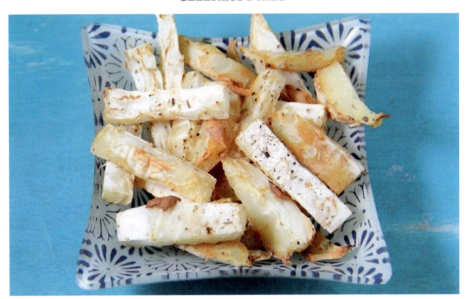

Preparation Time: 5 Minutes
Cooking Time: 10 Minutes
Servings: 3

Ingredients:

- Mixed Herbs, dried-2 teaspoons
- Celeriac, washed & cut into strips-1
- Dash of Chili flakes
- Rosemary Sprigs, stripped-4
- Salt -1/2 teaspoon
- Black Pepper, as desired

Method of Preparation:

1. To make these scrumptious celeriac fries, you need to preheat the oven to 400°F.
2. Put the celeriac in a pot of boiling water over medium-high heat.
3. Once the water starts boiling, remove the celeriac from the water. Drain it well.

4. Arrange the pieces on a baking sheet and top them with olive oil, chili flakes, salt, dried herbs and rosemary. Coat well.
5. Roast them for 40 to 45 minutes or until the insides are squishy and exteriors are crispy. Tip: Take them out once in between and flip them over.
6. Serve them hot.

Tip: Instead of cutting, you can also make wedges out of the celeriac.

Nutritional Information per serving:

- Calories: 18 Kcal
- Carbohydrates: 3.7 g
- Fat: 0.3 g
- Proteins: 0.5 g

10 Vegan Soups

Turmeric & Lentil Soup

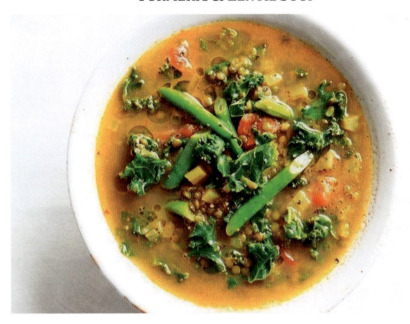

Preparation Time: 15 Minutes
Cooking Time: 50 Minutes
Servings: 2

Ingredients:

- Olive Oil -2 tablespoons
- Mustard Seeds-1 teaspoon
- Water-1 1/2 cups
- Garlic cloves, peeled & minced-3
- Cumin -1 teaspoon
- Red Lentils, split-1/4 cup
- Turmeric-1 teaspoon
- Carrots, organic, peeled & sliced-6
- Mixed Herbs -1 tablespoon
- Coconut Milk -6 tablespoons

For the beans:
- Garlic cloves-2
- Canned Cannellini Beans -1 (29 oz.)
- Dried Herbs -1 tablespoon
- Cremini/crimini mushroom Mushrooms -12

Method of Preparation:

1. Place the sliced carrots onto a parchment lined baking sheet.
2. Sprinkle the mixed herbs, pepper, salt and olive oil over them and toss well.
3. Place them into the oven and cook for 25 minutes at 350 degree or until soft and tender.
4. In the meantime, cook the lentils in a small pot of water over medium-high heat for 10 minutes and then simmer for another couple of minutes.
5. Heat the oil in a skillet over medium heat and add the mustard seeds, cumin and turmeric powder.
6. Place the lentil mixture and carrots into a high-speed blender and blend for about 30 to 40 seconds or until you have a purée.
7. Transfer the mustard seed mixture to a large bowl and add the purée. Stir well.
8. Serve it hot

Tip: For added kick if you like, you can use paprika.

Nutritional Information per serving:

- Calories: 336 Kcal
- Carbohydrates: 37 g
- Fat:17.3 g
- Proteins: 10.9 g

Roasted Tomato Soup

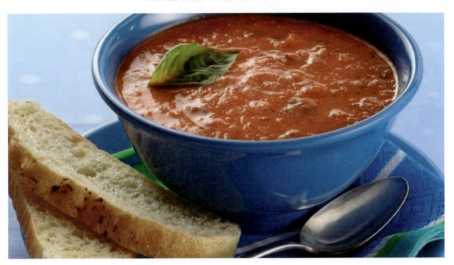

Preparation Time: 10 Minutes
Cooking Time: 60 Minutes
Servings: 4

Ingredients:

- Thyme, dried-1 teaspoon
- Vegetable Broth-3 cups
- Olive Oil -1 teaspoon
- Potato, medium, peeled & chopped -1
- Rosemary, fresh & diced-1 tablespoon
- Garlic cloves -4
- Can of Tomatoes, sliced lengthwise -1 (28 ounces)
- Cauliflower head, rinsed & chopped to florets -1/2
- Sea Salt, as desired
- Yellow Onion, medium & chopped finely-1/2
- Black Pepper, as desired

Method of Preparation:

1. Preheat the oven to 350°F.

2. Grease a baking sheet with olive oil and place the tomatoes on it with the cut side down on one end of the baking sheet. Reserve a cup of the tomato juice.
3. Place the garlic cloves also on the baking sheet near the tomatoes.
4. Sprinkle salt over the tomatoes and garlic. Bake them for 25 or 30 minutes or until the tomatoes are roasted.
5. Mix together the cauliflower, potatoes and onion in a mixing bowl along with the remaining oil, thyme, rosemary, pepper and salt.
6. Once the tomatoes are roasted, remove from the sheet and arrange the seasoned vegetables on the baking sheet.
7. Roast them for 25-30 minutes or until the vegetables are tender.
8. Take the sheet from the oven and let the vegetables cool.
9. Place them all in a high-speed blender and blend them for a few minutes or until the mixture becomes a smooth soup.
10. Transfer the soup to a pot and heat it over low heat until the soup is warm.
11. Add the remaining tomato juice and stir again.
12. Serve it hot.

Tip: If you want a thinner soup, you can add ½ cup of vegetable broth.

Nutritional Information per serving:

- Calories: 101 Kcal
- Carbohydrates: 14.9 g
- Fat: 2.5 g
- Proteins: 6 g

Sweet Potato Soup

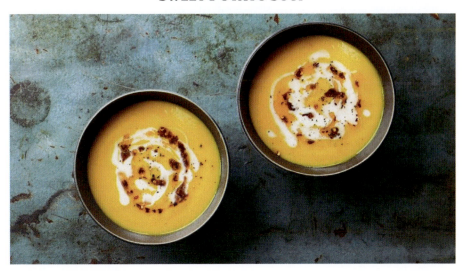

Preparation Time: 10 Minutes
Cooking Time: 50 Minutes
Servings: 2

Ingredients:

- Nut Milk, unsweetened-1/2 cup
- Sweet Potato, medium -1
- Lime juice-2 tablespoons
- Chipotle Pepper, seeded and chopped-1/4 teaspoon
- Vegetable Broth -1 cup
- clove of Garlic -1

Method of Preparation:

1. Preheat the oven to 400°F.
2. Use a fork, poke holes in the potato and bake it for about one hour on a baking sheet or until the sweet potato becomes tender.
3. When the potato is cool, remove the skin.

4. Place the cooked sweet potato and all the remaining ingredients in a high-speed blender and blend for 2 to 3 minutes or until you get a smooth soup.
5. Check for seasoning and correct as needed.
6. Finally, transfer the soup to a pot and heat it over low heat until the soup is warm.
7. Top it with your choice of toppings such as avocado or a sprinkle of paprika.

Tip: For more flavor, you can add cayenne or cumin.

Nutritional Information per serving:

- Calories: 81 Kcal
- Carbohydrates: 13.1 g
- Fat: 1.4 g
- Proteins: 3.9 g

BROCCOLI BISQUE

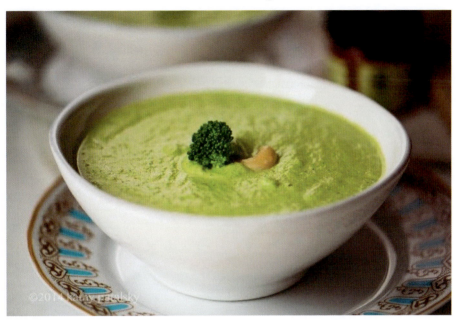

Preparation Time: 5 Minutes
Cooking Time: 15 Minutes + Soaking Time
Servings: 2

Ingredients:

- Vegetable Broth -2 cups
- Cashews, soaked overnight, drained & rinsed-3/4 cup
- Broccoli florets-3 cups

Method of Preparation:

1. Steam the broccoli in a steamer for 6 to 7 minutes or until softened and tender.
2. Place the cashews, broccoli and vegetable broth in a high-speed blender and blend until the mixture becomes a smooth soup.
3. Finally, transfer the soup to a small pot and simmer it over low heat.

4. Serve it hot.

Tip: You can add 1 to 2 tablespoons nutritional yeast for a cheesy flavor.

Nutritional Information per serving:

- Calories: 358 Kcal
- Carbohydrates: 25.6g
- Fat: 23.1 g
- Proteins: 17.5 g

BLACK BEAN SOUP

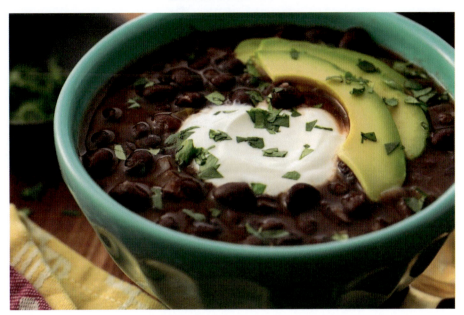

Preparation Time: 10 Minutes
Cooking Time: 1 Hour
Servings: 6

Ingredients:

- Cumin -2 teaspoons
- Black Beans, dried & rinsed-1 pound
- Salsa-1 cup
- Onion, large & diced-1
- Corn Kernels-12 ounces
- Water, boiling -6 cups
- Chipotle Chile Powder-1/4 teaspoon

Method of Preparation:

1. Boil the water in a pot over medium heat.
2. Press the 'sauté' button on an Instant Pot and add a small amount of oil.
3. Stir in the onion and cook until it is translucent.

4. Pour the boiling water into the pot along with chipotle powder, beans, salt and cumin. Mix well.
5. Turn off the 'sauté' button and lock the lid.
6. Once locked, press the 'manual' button and cook for 30 minutes on high pressure.
7. After half an hour, allow the pressure to release naturally.
8. Open the lid and check the beans for doneness. If not fully cooked, cook for another 2 minutes on high pressure.
9. Place half the cooked beans in a food processor and blend them into a purée.
10. Finally, return the beand to the soup in the pot. Add the corn and salsa.
11. Give everything a good stir and check for seasoning. Add more of the seasoning if needed.
12. Press the 'sauté' button again and cook until it is hot while stirring frequently.

Tip: Garnish it with avocado and soy yoghurt.

Nutritional Information per serving:

- Calories: 329 Kcal
- Carbohydrates: 65 g
- Fat: 1 g
- Proteins: 18 g

Creamy Asparagus Soup

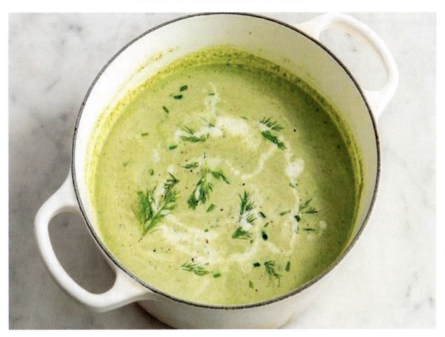

Preparation Time: 10 Minutes
Cooking Time: 25 Minutes
Servings: 4

Ingredients:

- Asparagus, trimmed -2 lb
- White Pepper-1/8 teaspoon
- Garlic cloves, minced-2
- Cashews, raw-1/2 pound
- Onion, small & sliced -1/2
- Vegetable Broth -2 cups
- Zest of Lemon-1/2
- Sea Salt, as desired
- Black Pepper, as desired

Method of Preparation:

1. Preheat the oven to 450°F.

2. Place the asparagus spears on a parchment lined baking sheet and roast them for 10 minutes.
3. Remove them from the oven and flip them over. Top the spears with onion and garlic.
4. Roast them again for another 10 minutes or until the veggies are tender.
5. In the meantime, place the cashews, half the vegetable broth and the pepper in a blender and blend for a few minutes or until it becomes smooth.
6. Once the asparagus are cooked, remove the tops from some of the spears and use them as a garnish later on.
7. Cut the remaining spears into pieces.
8. Add the spears, onion and garlic along with the remaining vegetable broth into the blender and blend until smooth and creamy.
9. Transfer the soup to a pot and simmer until warm.
10. Garnish it with the lemon zest and the remaining spear tops.

Tip: Instead of raw cashews, you can also use cashew butter.

Nutritional Information per serving:

- Calories: 76 kcal
- Carbohydrates: 12.4 g
- Fat: 1.96 g
- Proteins: 6.4 g

Arugula Artichoke Soup

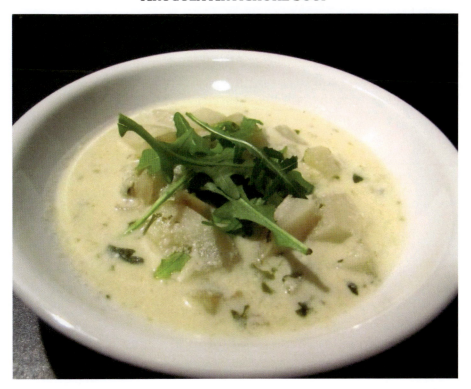

Preparation Time: 15 Minutes
Cooking Time: 25 Minutes
Servings: 2

Ingredients:

- Baby Arugula -1 1/2 cups
- Garlic, finely minced-3 cloves
- Vegetable Broth-1 1/2 cups
- Black Pepper-1/4 teaspoon
- White Onion, finely diced-1
- Sea Salt-1 teaspoon
- Artichoke Hearts, drained & chopped-6 oz
- Lemon Juice, fresh -2 tablespoons
- Tofu, firm -1 cup

Method of Preparation:

1. Add vegetable broth (a small amount) to a pot and heat it over medium-high heat.
2. Once the broth is hot, stir in the onion and garlic, and cook for 3 to 4 minutes or until the onion is soft.
3. Add the artichoke hearts to the pot and cook for another five minutes, covered.
4. Place the tofu and half the vegetable broth in a food processor and blend until it becomes a smooth purée.
5. Spoon the artichoke mixture into the food process and pulse until you get a chunky soup.
6. Transfer the soup back to the pot and stir in the arugula, nutritional yeast and lemon juice.
7. Finally, add the remaining vegetable broth until you obtain the desired consistency.
8. Check for seasoning and add more salt and pepper, if needed.

Tip: If you prefer a smooth soup, you can blend it fully without leaving any chunks.

Nutritional Information per serving:

- ➢ Calories: 382 kcal
- ➢ Carbohydrates: 61.6 g
- ➢ Fat: 7.3 g
- ➢ Proteins: 31.3 g

Cauliflower Tomato Soup

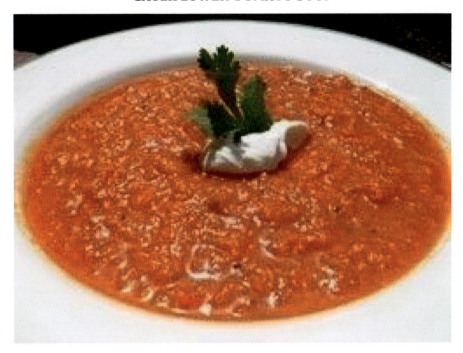

Preparation Time: 5 Minutes
Cooking Time: 40 Minutes
Servings: 6

Ingredients:

- Swiss Chard, chopped-2 cups
- Cauliflower head -2 pounds
- Red Pepper, crushed -1/4 teaspoon
- Olive Oil -1/2 tablespoon
- Sea Salt -1/4 teaspoon
- Carrot, diced-1/2
- Italian Seasoning, dried -1 teaspoon
- White Onion, diced-1
- Chickpeas, cooked -1 can (15 ounces)
- Vegetable Broth -2 cups
- Cauliflower Head, florets, washed-2 pounds (florets)
- Tomato Sauce-1 can (15 ounces)

- Pinch of Black Pepper
- Diced Tomatoes -1 can (15 ounces)

Method of Preparation:

1. Preheat the oven to 375° F.
2. Place the florets, pepper, salt and olive oil in a large mixing bowl. Toss well.
3. Put on a parchment paper-lined baking sheet and bake for 25 to 30 minutes.
4. Stir the cauliflower once while baking. In the meantime, heat the vegetable broth in a pot over medium heat.
5. Once the broth is hot, stir in the onion and cook for 4 to 5 minutes or until softened.
6. Add the diced tomatoes, tomato sauce, carrot, chickpeas and the remaining vegetable broth.
7. Bring the mixture to a boil. Lower the heat and let it simmer.
8. As it is simmering, stir in the chickpeas, red pepper flakes and Italian seasoning. Mix well.
9. Finally, add the cauliflower florets and stir well until everything is well combined. Cover the pot and simmer for five minutes before serving.

Tip: To make it thinner, you can add more vegetable broth.

Nutritional Information per serving:

- Calories: 102 Kcal
- Carbohydrates: 16.8 g
- Fat: 2.1 g
- Proteins: 5.3 g

Curried Corn Chowder

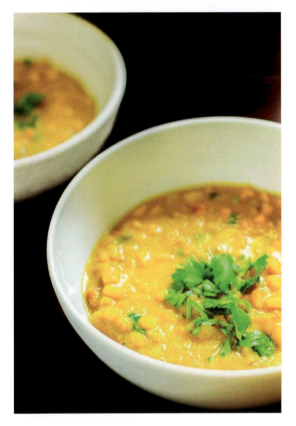

Preparation Time: 5 Minutes
Cooking Time: 25 Minutes
Servings: 6

Ingredients:

- Garlic cloves, minced-3
- Coconut Milk -2 cups (16 ounces)
- Yellow Onion, finely diced-1
- Olive Oil -1 tablespoon
- Corn, fresh -3 1/2 ounces
- Ginger, grated -1 tablespoon
- Vegetable Broth -4 cups
- Sugar -1/2 teaspoon

- Salt -1/2 teaspoon
- Curry Powder- 1 tablespoon
- Black Pepper, to taste

Method of Preparation:

1. Heat the oil in a pot of a large size over medium heat.
2. Once the oil is hot, stir in the onions and cook for 3 to 4 minutes or until softened.
3. Stir in the garlic, sugar and ginger. Cook for 4 minutes or until browned.
4. Add the curry powder to the garlic mix and stir for a minute.
5. Pour in the vegetable broth and mix until everything is blended.
6. Add the corn and combine well.
7. Allow the soup to simmer for about 5 to 6 minutes. Set it aside to cool.
8. Once slightly cool, purée the mixture in a food processor or with an immersion blender until it becomes smooth.
9. Finally, return the soup to the pot and add the coconut milk.
10. Cook for another 8 to 10 minutes over low heat.
11. Check for seasoning and correct if needed.
12. Serve it hot.

Tip: If desired, you can garnish it with cilantro.

Nutritional Information per serving:

- ➢ Calories: 293 Kcal
- ➢ Carbohydrates: 25.3 g
- ➢ Fat: 20.3 g
- ➢ Proteins: 8.2g

CARROT SOUP

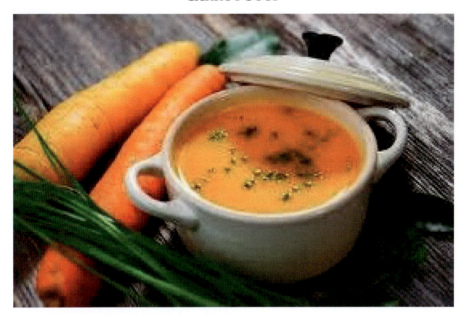

Preparation Time: 10 Minutes
Cooking Time: 40 Minutes
Servings: 6

Ingredients:

- Vegetable Broth -1 1/2 cups
- Juice of Lemon-1
- Onion, medium & chopped-1
- Cashews, chopped-1/2 cup
- Canola Oil -1 tablespoon
- Pinch of Red Chili Flakes
- Ginger, fresh & chopped-1 tablespoon
- Coconut Milk -2 cups (16 ounces)
- Tamari -1 tablespoon
- Carrots, medium & diced-5

Method of Preparation:

1. Heat the oil in a saucepan of a large size over medium heat.

2. Add the onions and cook for 3 to 4 minutes or until softened.
3. Stir in the red chili flakes, ginger, carrots and tamari. Cook for 2 minutes.
4. Pour the broth and coconut milk into it and bring the mixture to a boil.
5. Reduce the heat, then let it simmer.
6. Simmer for 18 or 20 minutes or until the carrots are soft.
7. Check for seasoning and correct if needed. In the meantime, mix together lime juice, cashews, salt and cilantro in a bowl.
8. Finally, place the carrot mixture in a blender and purée until it becomes smooth.
9. Transfer the purée to the serving bowls and top with the cashew sauce.

Tip: Instead of red chili flakes, you can also use chili garlic sauce.

Nutritional Information per serving:

- Calories: 283 Kcal
- Carbohydrates: 15.4 g
- Fat: 23.9 g
- Proteins: 5.6 g

10 Vegan Main Meals

Vegan Banana Bread

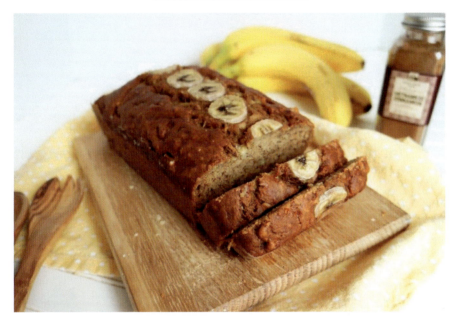

Preparation Time: 10 Minutes
Cooking Time: 50 Minutes
Servings: 1 Loaf

Ingredients:

Wet ingredients:
- Bananas, organic, ripe & mashed -4
- Vanilla Extract -2 teaspoons
- Almond Milk -1/3 cup
- Flax Seeds, ground-2 tablespoons
- Vanilla Extract, pure -2 teaspoons
- Coconut Oil -1/3 cup
- Maple Syrup -2 tablespoons

Dry ingredients:
- Sea Salt-1/2 teaspoon
- Coconut Sugar -1/4 cup +2 tablespoons

- Baking Soda- 1 teaspoon
- Rolled Oats -1/2 cup
- White Spelt Flour -1 1/2 cups
- Baking Powder-1/2 teaspoon

Method of Preparation:

1. Preheat the oven to 350°F.
2. Place the bananas in a mixing bowl and mash them well.
3. Add all the wet ingredients to the bowl and stir the mixture until everything is well combined.
4. Stir in all the dry ingredients. Mix well until there are no more lumps.
5. Once everything has come together, grease a loaf pan with oil.
6. Spoon the batter into the pan and spread it to the sides evenly.
7. Bake it for 40 to 45 minutes or until the top is lightly golden and firm.
8. Remove the bread from the oven and allow it to cool completely before removing if from the pan and slicing.

Tip: You can use toppings like chopped walnuts or chocolate chips if desired.

Nutritional Information per serving:

- Calories: 190 Kcal
- Carbohydrates: 29 g
- Fat: 7 g
- Proteins: 3 g

Chickpea Omelet

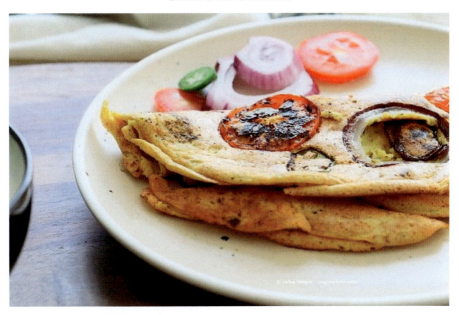

Preparation Time: 10 Minutes
Cooking Time: 20 Minutes
Servings: 1

Ingredients:

- Spinach, fresh -1/4 cup
- Flax Meal -1 tablespoon
- Baking Powder-1/2 teaspoon
- Oat Flour-1/2 tablespoon
- Jalapeño, chopped finely -1/2
- Chickpea Flour -1/3 cup
- Veggies (Onion, Tomato, etc.)-1/2 cup
- Garlic Powder-1/8 teaspoon
- Water -1 cup
- Pinch of Turmeric

Method of Preparation:

1. Combine flax meal and water (1/2 cup) in a medium-sized mixing bowl.
2. Whisk it well and allow it to sit for 10 minutes.
3. Spoon in the baking powder and then the chickpea flour, spices, oat flour, salt and the remaining water into the bowl.
4. Mix them until everything is combined and the batter is airy.
5. Stir in the veggies and jalapeño. Fold together well.
6. Heat a large pan over medium-high heat. Apply a bit of oil.
7. With a help of a scoop, spoon the batter into the pan and spread it out.
8. Cover the pan and cook it for 5 to 7 minutes until the batter is set.
9. Finally, flip it over once and cook for another 4 to 5 minutes.

Tip: You can pair it with more veggies and hash browns for a complete meal.

Nutritional Information per serving:

- Calories: 251 Kcal
- Carbohydrates: 36 g
- Fat: 6 g
- Proteins: 12 g

VEGAN PANCAKES

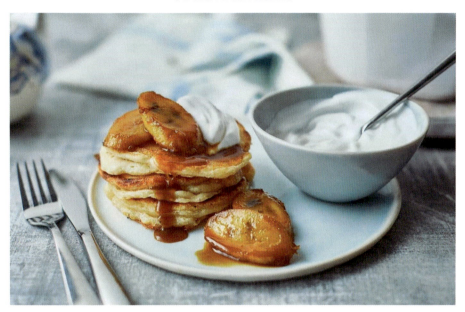

Preparation Time: 5 Minutes
Cooking Time: 10 Minutes
Servings: 12 pancakes

Ingredients:

- Almond Milk, unsweetened -1 1/2 cup
- Whole Wheat Pastry Flour -1 1/2 cups
- Coconut Oil -1 teaspoon
- Baking Powder-1 tablespoon
- Flax Egg (1 tablespoon flax seeds + 3 tablespoons water)-1
- Salt-1/2 teaspoon
- Vanilla Extract -1/2 teaspoon

Method of Preparation:

1. Soak the flax seeds in the water in a small bowl for about 10 minutes and set it aside.

2. Take the flour, salt and baking powder and sift them into a large mixing bowl.
3. Stir the almond milk, flax egg, vanilla, and coconut oil into the bowl. Whisk them well.
4. Once well combined, heat a large pan over medium heat.
5. Grease the pan with coconut oil and spoon the pancake batter into the pan letting the batter spread out before adding the next spoonful.
6. Cook them for 2 to 3 minutes per side.
7. Finally, serve it with your favorite topping.

Tip: Instead of whole wheat flour, you can also use spelt flour.

Nutritional Information per serving:

- Calories: 105 Kcal
- Carbohydrates: 14.4 g
- Fat: 3.6 g
- Proteins: 3.6 g

TOFU SCRAMBLE

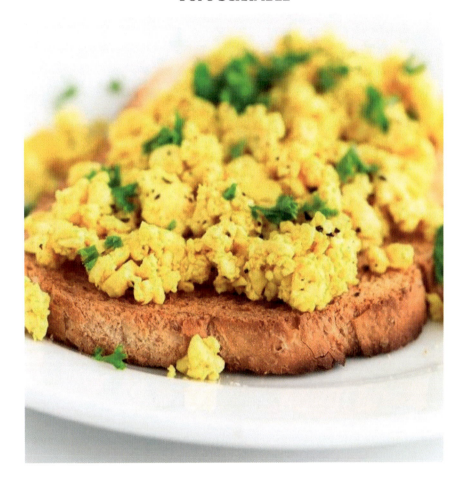

Preparation Time: 10 Minutes
Cooking Time: 10 Minutes
Servings: 2

Ingredients:

- Tofu, extra-firm -8 ounces
- Onion Powder-1/4 teaspoon
- Earth Balance Vegan Butter – 1 tablespoon
- Soy Milk -1/3 cup
- Nutritional Yeast -2 tablespoons

- Dijon Mustard -1/2 teaspoon
- Turmeric -1/2 teaspoon
- Salt -1/4 teaspoon
- Paprika -1/2 teaspoon

Method of Preparation:

1. Place the tofu in a bowl, mash it with a fork leaving a few chunky pieces.
2. Combine all the remaining ingredients, excluding the soy milk, in another bowl until mixed well.
3. Pour the soy milk into the bowl and whisk until you get a smooth mixture .
4. Melt the vegan butter in a heated pan over medium heat.
5. Once melted, stir in the tofu and sauté until it is lightly browned and cooked. Make sure not to break it up much while stirring.
6. Spoon the sauce into the pan and fold in the tofu.
7. Continue cooking until the scrambled tofu gets the desired consistency you want.
8. Finally, remove it from the heat and transfer to a serving bowl.
9. Serve it hot along with sliced avocado.

Tip: If you prefer, you can garnish it with black pepper and chives.

Nutritional Information per serving:

- Calories: 206Kcal
- Carbohydrates: 3.8g
- Fat: 13.1g
- Proteins: 20.3g

CHICKPEA PATTIES

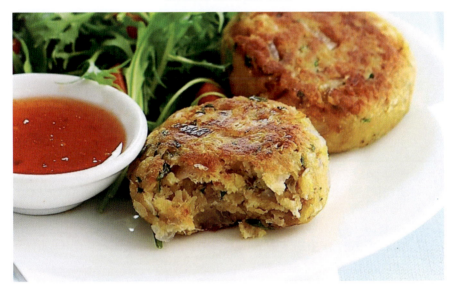

Preparation Time: 10 Minutes
Cooking Time: 30 Minutes
Servings: 8

Ingredients:

- Oats, crushed -1/2 cup
- Olive Oil – 1 tablespoon
- Beet, medium & grated -1/2
- Chili Powder-1/4 teaspoon
- Chickpeas, washed, drained & cooked-1/2 cup
- Cajun Seasoning -1/2 teaspoon
- Potato, medium & boiled-1/2
- Salt-1/2 teaspoon
- Garlic, minced-2 teaspoons
- Tomato Paste -1 tablespoon
- Cumin Powder-1/2 teaspoon

Method of Preparation:

1. Combine potato, beet and chickpeas in a large mixing bowl until well mixed.
2. Add spices, salt, tomato paste and olive oil and mix again until well incorporated.
3. Allow it to sit for 5 minutes and stir in about half the quantity of oats. Combine well. You can add more oats if needed to make it a dough.
4. Once it becomes a doughy consistency, make balls out of it and smash them into patties.
5. Immerse the patties into the remaining oats and coat both sides.
6. Place the patties on a parchment-lined baking sheet and bake them at 350°F for 15 to 20 minutes or until the patties becomes slightly crisp and browned.

Tip: Serve it along with greens or as sliders.

Nutritional Information per serving:

- Calories: 65 Kcal
- Carbohydrates: 9 g
- Fat: 2 g
- Proteins: 2 g

COCONUT CURRY

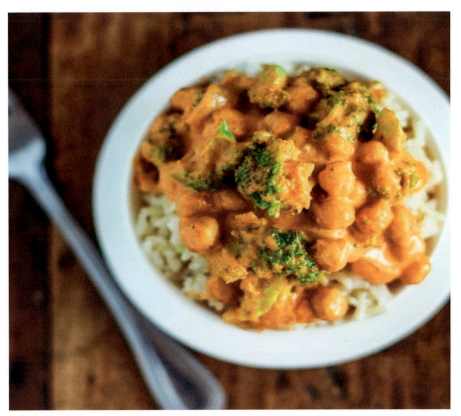

Preparation Time: 5 Minutes
Cooking Time: 5 Minutes
Serving Sizs: 4

Ingredients:

- Coconut milk – 1 can (14 oz.)
- Red curry paste – 2 tablespoons
- Chickpeas – 1 can (15 oz.)rinsed
- Broccoli heads – 2 small
- Cornstarch dissolved in water– 2 tablespoons
- Minced garlic, optional
- Olive oil – 1 tablespoon

Instructions

1. Sauté the broccoli with the garlic in olive oil for a few minutes. Add coconut milk and allow to simmer for about 8 minutes or until broccoli is soft and tender.
2. Add curry paste to the pan and whisk until well combined. Add chickpeas and bring to boil.
3. Add cornstarch and cook for a minute, and then remove from the heat and allow to cool.
4. Serve and enjoy

Tip: You can also substitute the garlic with onion if preferred.

Nutritional Information per serving:

- Calories: 518 Kcal
- Carbohydrates: 57.6 g
- Fat: 26.2 g
- Proteins: 19.1 g

Spinach-Parmesan Casserole

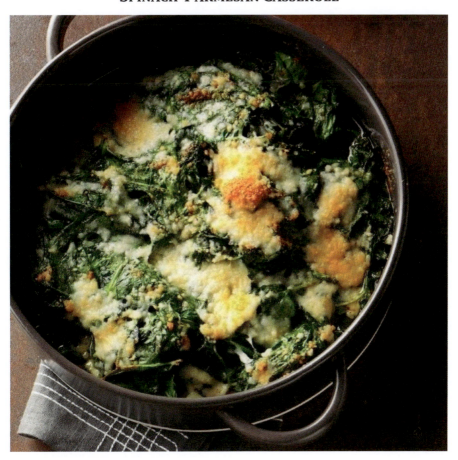

Preparation Time: 5 Minutes
Cooking Time: 18 Minutes
Servings: 6

Ingredients:

- Fresh baby spinach – 2 pounds
- Unsalted butter – 5 tablespoons
- Olive oil – 3 tablespoons
- Minced garlic cloves – 3
- Italian seasoning – 1 tablespoon
- Salt – ¾ teaspoon

- Grated parmesan cheese, vegan – 1 cup

Instructions

1. Preheat the oven to 400^0F
2. Add about 5 cups of water into a stockpot and bring to a boil. Add the spinach and cook for a minute or so until wilted. Drain well.
3. In a skillet heat oil and butter over medium heat. Add the Italian seasoning, garlic and salt. Cook for about two minutes as you stir.
4. Spread spinach into a greased baking dish and drizzle with the butter mixture. Sprinkle with the cheese and bake uncovered for 15 minutes or until cheese is browned.

Tip: You can also try sautéing the spinach instead of boiling it.

Nutritional Information per serving:

- ➢ Calories: 239 Kcal
- ➢ Carbohydrates: 7 g
- ➢ Fat: 21 g
- ➢ Proteins: 10 g

Spanakopita Mashed Potatoes

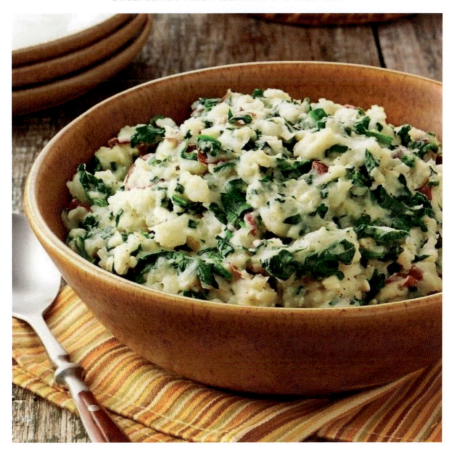

Preparation Time: 10 Minutes
Cooking Time: 25 Minutes
Servings: 6

Ingredients:

- Red potatoes quartered – 6 medium
- Fresh baby spinach – 1 package (6 ounces)
- Cowmilk – ¼ cup
- Butter – 1 tablespoon
- Salt and pepper – ½ teaspoon
- Crumbled feta cheese, (vegan) – ¾ cup

Method of Preparation:

1. Put the potatoes into a large saucepan. Cover with water and cook for 20 minutes or until the potatoes are tender.
2. In another large saucepan add 1/2 cup of water then bring it to a boil. Add the spinach, cover and allow to boil for 3 minutes. Once cooked, drain, remove from the pan and chop. Keep warm.
3. Drain the potatoes. Then place them back into the saucepan. Add butter, salt, milk and pepper and mash with the potatoes until well blended.
4. Fold in spinach and cheese, and serve warm.

Tip: The leftovers can be used for potato pancakes.

Nutritional Information per serving:

- Calories: 145 Kcal
- Carbohydrates: 20 g
- Fat: 5 g
- Proteins: 6 g

Tomato & Garlic Butter Beans

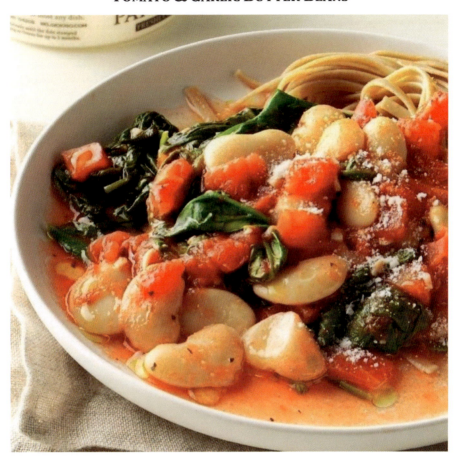

Preparation Time: 10 Minutes
Cooking Time: 10 Minutes
Servings: 4

Ingredients:

- Olive oil – 1 tablespoon
- Minced garlic cloves – 2
- Diced tomatoes, undrained – 2 cans (14.5 Oz.)
- Butter beans, rinsed and drained – 1 can (15 oz.)
- Fresh baby spinach – 6 cups
- Italian seasoning – ½ teaspoon

- Black Pepper – ½ teaspoon
- Grated parmesan cheese, vegan – optional

Method of Preparation:

1. In a skillet, add oil and heat over medium heat. Add garlic, stir and cook for about 45 seconds.
2. Add beans, tomatoes, Italian seasoning, spinach and pepper. Cook for about 5 or 6 minutes or until the spinach is wilted.
3. You can serve it once ready with cheese or pasta.

Tip: The leftovers can be used as potato pancakes.

Nutritional Information per serving:

- Calories: 147 Kcal
- Carbohydrates: 28 g
- Fat: 4 g
- Proteins: 8 g

Spanish Spinach with Chickpeas

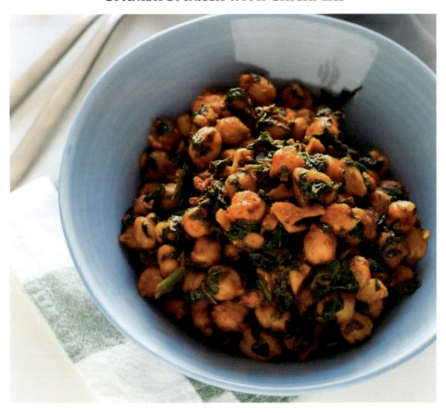

Preparation Time: 5 Minutes
Cooking Time: 15 Minutes
Servings: 4

Ingredients:

- Olive oil – 2 tablespoons
- Garlic Cloves, diced – 1 head
- Spinach – 1 cup
- Water – ½ cup
- Cooked chickpeas – 3½ cups
- Sea salt
- Sweet paprika – 3 tablespoons

Method of Preparation:

1. In a saucepan cook diced garlic with a tablespoon of olive oil over medium heat until golden brown, then add paprika and stir.
2. Add spinach and water and cook for 5 minutes. Add salt and stir. You can also use oil to cook the spinach instead of water.
3. Add the cooked chickpeas to the saucepan and stir. Add another spoon of olive oil and cook for 5 more minutes.
4. Serve immediately

Tip: You can substitute spinach with your preferred vegetables. However, spinach with chickpeas is a known Spanish traditional recipe which is loved by many.

Nutritional Information per serving:

- Calories: 209 Kcal
- Carbohydrates: 28 g
- Fat: 8 g
- Proteins: 7 g

10 Vegan Desserts

Golden Milk Smoothie

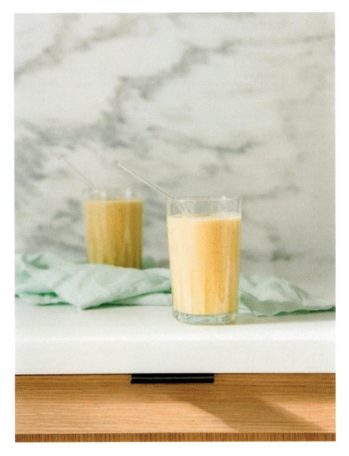

Preparation Time: 5 Minutes
Cooking Time: 3 Minutes
Servings: 1

Ingredients:

- Banana, ripe, sliced & frozen -1 cup
- Carrot Juice, fresh -1/4 cup
- Coconut Milk, light – 1 cup

- Dash of Black Pepper
- Turmeric Powder-1/2 teaspoon
- Dash of Cinnamon, ground
- Ginger, fresh -1 tablespoon
- Hemp Seed-1 tablespoon
- A pinch of Nutmeg, ground

Method of Preparation:

1. For making this lip-smacking smoothie, place the banana in a high-speed blender and then add coconut milk, ginger, turmeric, cinnamon, black pepper, and nutmeg to it.
2. Close the lid and blend for 3 to 4 minutes or until the mixture becomes smooth and rich.
3. If the smoothie seems too thick, add more coconut milk and mix well.
4. Finally, transfer the luxurious smoothie to a serving glass and serve it immediately.

Tip: If you prefer to have a spicier taste and texture, you can add clove and cardamom to it.

Nutritional Information per serving:

- Calories: 295 Kcal
- Carbohydrates: 43.7 g
- Fat: 4.6 g
- Proteins: 3.5 g

Strawberry Chia Pudding

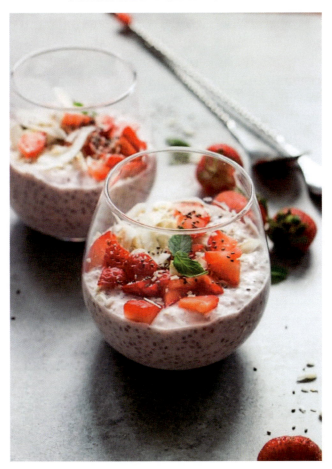

Preparation Time: 5 Minutes
Cooking Time: 15 Minutes
Servings: 2

Ingredients:

- Almond Milk -1 1/2 cups
- Medjool Dates, pitted-2
- Chia Seeds-1 tablespoons
- Ginger, fresh & grated-2 teaspoons
- Strawberries, fresh-1 cup

Method of Preparation:

1. Place the strawberries, dates, almond milk and ginger in a high-speed blender and blend for about 2 to 3 minutes or until the mixture becomes smooth & silky.
2. Put the mixture into a mixing bowl. Add all the chia seeds. Stir well.
3. Allow the mixture to sit for 8 to 10 minutes or until it has a pudding consistency.
4. Place it in the refrigerator until ready to be served.

Tip: Top it with strawberries if desired.

Nutritional Information per serving:

- Calories: 201 Kcal
- Carbohydrates: 39.3 g
- Fat: 4.64 g
- Proteins: 2.82 g

Sweet Potato Oatmeal

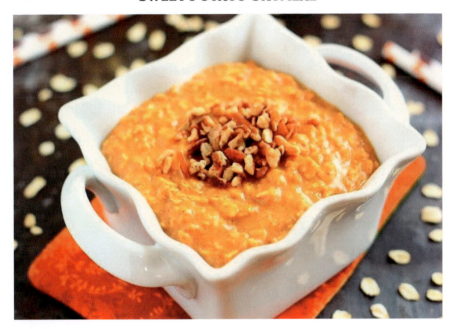

Preparation Time: 5 Minutes
Cooking Time: 25 Minutes
Servings: 3

Ingredients:

- Rolled Oats -1 cup
- Flax Seed Meal -1/2 tablespoon
- Water -1 3/4 cups
- Maple Syrup -2 tablespoons
- Sweet Potato-1 large
- Cinnamon, ground-1/2 teaspoon
- Pecans, roasted -3 tablespoons

Method of Preparation:

1. For making this delicious fall inspired oatmeal porridge, you need to slice a sweet potato into 2 halves and then apply olive oil lightly over it.

2. Place the sweet potato with flesh side down on a parchment-lined baking sheet and bake at 350 degrees for 23 to 25 minutes or until soft.
3. Boil the water in a deep saucepan over medium heat.
4. Once it starts boiling, stir in the oats and reduce the heat to low.
5. Continue cooking for 4 minutes or until all the water has been absorbed while stirring frequently.
6. In the meantime, remove the sweet potato from the oven and mash it with a spoon or fork until it is a smooth purée. Set aside.
7. Add the sweet potato purée, flax seed meal, maple syrup, and cinnamon to the saucepan with the oats. Mix them well.
8. Check for sweetness. Add more syrup if needed. If the oats seem too thick, you can add a splash of nut milk to them.
9. Finally, transfer the oatmeal to a serving bowl and top with pecans.

Tip: Instead of maple syrup, you can use brown sugar.

Nutritional Information per serving:

- Calories: 253 Kcal
- Carbohydrates: 55.9 g
- Fat: 8.8 g
- Proteins: 9.7 g

Peanut Butter Oatmeal

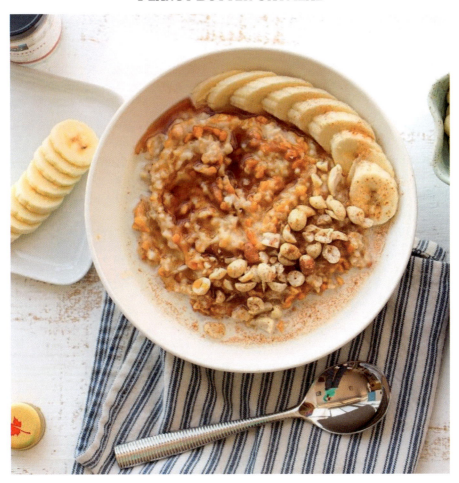

Preparation Time: 10 Minutes
Cooking Time: 15 Minutes
Servings: 4

Ingredients:

- Banana, organic-2
- Water -4 cups
- Cinnamon -1 teaspoon
- Steel Cut Oats -1 cup
- Peanuts, roasted, whole -2 tablespoons

- Salt -1/8 teaspoon
- Maple Syrup-3 tablespoons
- Peanut Butter -1/2 cup
- Nut Milk, to taste

Method of Preparation:

1. To make this easy oatmeal, you need to place the oats and water in a deep pan along with the salt.
2. Heat it over medium-high heat, cover and bring the mixture to a boil.
3. Reduce the heat to low and cook for 20 minutes or until the oats are creamy.
4. Stir together the peanut butter and 2 tablespoons of peanuts in a small bowl.
5. Microwave this mixture on high for 30 seconds or until you get a soft and melted butter.
6. Spoon half of the peanut butter into the oats and swirl it lightly.
7. Finally, transfer the oats to a serving bowl and add the remaining peanut butter mixture to it.
8. Mix until everything is well incorporated.
9. Garnish with the sliced bananas and maple syrup.

Tip: Instead of peanut butter, you can use cashew butter or almond butter.

Nutritional Information per serving:

- ➢ Calories: 428 Kcal
- ➢ Carbohydrates: 47
- ➢ Fat: 20 g
- ➢ Proteins: 15 g

CARROT CAKE OATMEAL

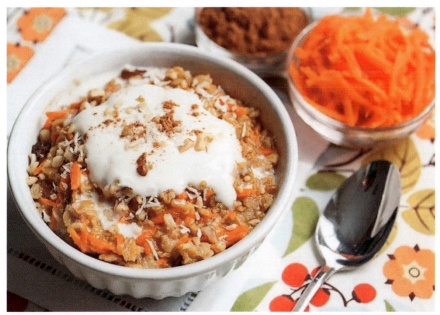

Preparation Time: 15 Minutes
Cooking Time: 10 Minutes
Servings: 2

Ingredients:

- Lemon Juice, fresh -1/4 teaspoon
- Carrot, grated -1 cup
- Vanilla Extract -1 teaspoon
- Cinnamon, ground-1 teaspoon
- Almond Milk, unsweetened -1 1/4 cups
- Rolled Oats -1/2 cup
- Maple Syrup -1 tablespoon +1 teaspoon
- Ginger, ground-1/4 teaspoon
- Pinch of Salt
- Dash of Nutmeg, ground

Method of Preparation:

1. Mix together the almond milk, nutmeg, maple syrup, salt, cinnamon, and ginger in a medium-size pot until well combined. Heat on high heat.
2. Stir in the carrot and oats. Combine well.
3. Bring the mixture to a boil and lower the heat to medium.
4. Once it starts simmering, cook, uncovered, for another 9 to 11 minutes or until the mixture is thickened.
5. Remove the pot and spoon in the vanilla extract. Stir again.
6. Pour it to a serving bowl and top it with your choice of toppings.

Tip: For toppings, you could consider chopped walnuts or shredded coconut or both.

Nutritional Information per serving:

- Calories: 200 Kcal
- Carbohydrates: 35 g
- Fat: 4 g
- Proteins: 5 g

Savory Oatmeal

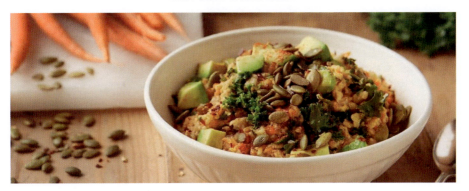

Preparation Time: 10 Minutes
Cooking Time: 20 Minutes
Servings: 4

Ingredients:

- Pine Nuts, roasted -1/4 cup
- Steel Cut Oats -1 cup
- White Onion, sliced thinly-1/2
- Vegetable Broth -2 cups
- Kale leaves, fresh, chopped-4 cups
- Shiitake Mushrooms, chopped-2 cups
- Water-1/2 cup
- Garlic cloves, minced-4
- Coconut Oil -1 tablespoon

Method of Preparation:

1. Combine the prepared vegetable broth and water in a medium saucepan and heat over medium heat.
2. Bring the mixture to a boil and add the oats.
3. Reduce the heat to low and cook them for 25 to 30 minutes or until the oats are cooked and the water has been absorbed.
4. In the meantime, heat the coconut oil in a large skillet over medium heat.

5. Once the oil is hot, stir in the onion and garlic.
6. Sauté them for 3 to 4 minutes or until aromatic.
7. Add the mushrooms and cook for another 5 to 6 minutes or until browned lightly.
8. Stir in the kale and sauté for 2 to 3 minutes or until the kale is wilted.
9. Transfer the cooked oats to serving bowls and top them with the kale-mushroom mixture and pine nuts. You can even add a fried egg on the top, if desired.

Tip: You can add your choice of veggies to this.

Nutritional Information per serving:

- Calories: 327 Kcal
- Carbohydrates: 44 g
- Fat: 13 g
- Proteins: 13 g

Mint-Chip Coconut Milk Ice Cream

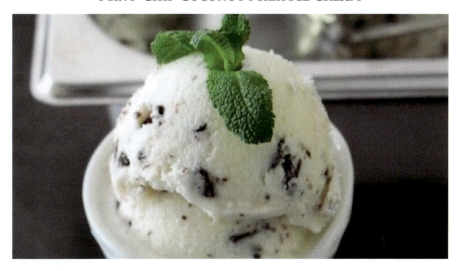

Preparation Time: 10 Minutes
Cooking Time: 2 hours 10 Minutes
Servings: 4

Ingredients:

- Coconut milk – 24 ounces
- Agave syrup to taste
- Peppermint extract to taste
- Dark chocolate chopped into pieces – 3 Ounces

Method of Preparation:

1. Chill all of the ingredients before preparing to shorten the freezing time.
2. Add coconut milk into a blender and blend well until smooth. Add peppermint extract and agave syrup to the blender and blend again.
3. Transfer the mixture to an ice cream maker. Follow the manufacturer's instructions to make the ice cream.
4. Add pieces of chocolate as desired and put it on your freezer for about 2 hours before serving.

Tip: The result is creamy and sweet

Nutritional Information per serving:

- Calories: 269 Kcal
- Carbohydrates: 19.4 g
- Fat: 22 g
- Proteins: 2.3 g

Vegan Chocolate Ice Cream

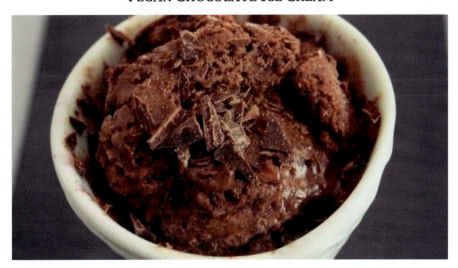

Preparation Time: 15 Minutes
Cooking Time: 5 Minutes
Servings: 4

Ingredients:

- Chopped dark chocolate – 7 ounces
- Aquafaba – 1 ¼ cups
- Xanthan gum – ½ teaspoon
- Confectioner's sugar – ½ cup
- Vanilla sugar – ½ cup

Method of Preparation:

1. Melt chopped dark chocolate over simmering water in a double boiler for 10 minutes. Stir frequently and scrape down the sides using a spatula to avoid scorching.
2. Pour aquafaba into a bowl and beat until fluffy, about one minute.
3. Add xanthan gum and beat for about 30 seconds. Add vanilla and confectioner's sugar.
4. Continue beating for about 2 minutes until the mixture becomes glossy and firm.

5. Fold melted chocolate into the whipped mixture until well incorporated. Transfer to a container with a lid.
6. Freeze the mixture overnight. Serve when desired.

Tip: The end result is a nice frozen mousse type of dessert.

Nutritional Information per serving:

- Calories: 180 Kcal
- Carbohydrates: 1.4 g
- Fat: 8 g
- Proteins: 1.4 g

ORANGE VEGAN CAKE

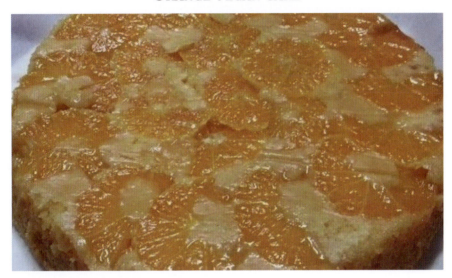

Preparation Time: 15 Minutes
Cooking Time: 30 Minutes
Servings: 6

Ingredients:

- Orange, Juiced – 1 cup
- All purpose flour – 1 ½ cups
- White sugar – 1 cup
- Vegetable oil – ½ cup
- Baking soda – 1½ teaspoons
- Salt – ¼ teaspoon

Method of Preparation:

1. Preheat the oven to 375°F. Grease a baking pan.
2. Blend orange in a blender until liquefied. Measure 1 cup of orange juice.
3. Whisk together the orange juice, sugar , vegetable oil, baking soda and salt in a large bowl and pour the mixture into the greased pan.

4. Bake the vegan cake in the preheated oven for about 30 minutes or until an inserted toothpick comes out clean.
5. Allow to cool and serve when desired.

Nutritional Information per serving:

- Calories: 157 Kcal
- Carbohydrates: 22.8 g
- Fat: 7 g
- Proteins: 1.3 g

Vegan Strawberry Oatmeal Smoothie

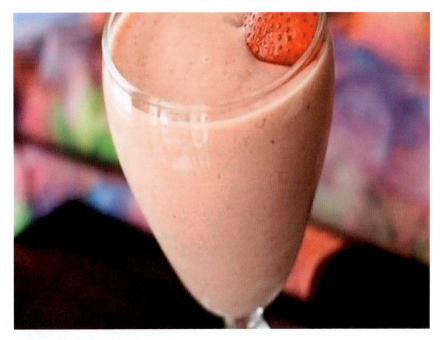

Preparation Time: 10 Minutes
Cooking Time: 10 Minutes
Servings: 2

Ingredients:

- Almond Milk – 1 cup
- Rolled oats – ½ cup
- Frozen strawberries – 14
- Banana broken into chunks – 1
- Agave nectar – 1½ teaspoons
- Vanilla extract – ½ teaspoon

Method of Preparation:

1. Blend strawberries, almond milk, oats, banana, agave nectar and vanilla extract together in a blender until smooth.

Tip: You can use rice milk if desired in place of almond milk.

Nutritional Information per serving:

- Calories: 205 Kcal
- Carbohydrates: 42.4 g
- Fat: 3 g
- Proteins: 4.2 g

10 Vegan Sauses

Kale Walnut Pesto

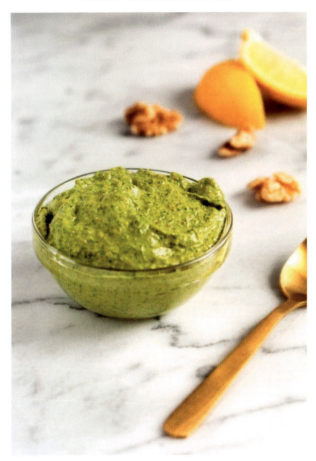

Preparation Time: 15 Minutes
Cooking Time: 5 Minutes
Servings: 1

Ingredients:

- Bunch of kale – ½, discard the stems, chop the leaves
- Chopped walnuts – ½ cup
- Cloves garlic – 2
- Nutritional yeast – ¼ cup

- Lemon juice – ½ lemon
- Olive oil – ¼ cup
- Salt and pepper to taste

Method of Preparation:

2. Place a large pot of water over medium heat and bring to a boil. Add salt and kale and cook for about 5 minutes.
3. Transfer the kale to a colander to drain and place in a blender. Combine with the garlic, walnuts, olive oil, nutritional yeast and lemon juice to taste.
4. Blend the mixture until smooth and taste for seasoning. Add more lemon juice and salt to taste, if needed.

Tip: This is a versatile sauce which is also great when used as a vegetable dip.

Nutritional Information per serving:

- Calories: 205 Kcal
- Carbohydrates: 42.4 g
- Fat: 3 g
- Proteins: 4.2 g

VEGAN RANCH DRESSING

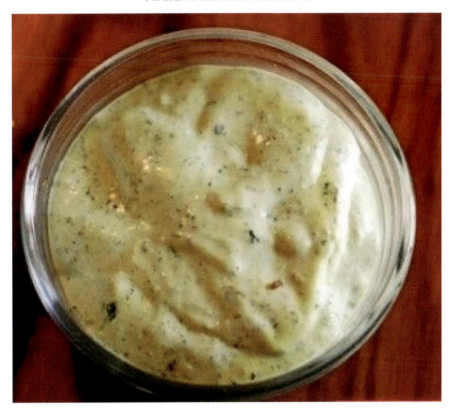

Preparation Time: 10 Minutes
Cooking Time: 5 Minutes
Servings: 2

Ingredients:

- Vegan mayonnaise – 1 cup
- Garlic powder – ½ teaspoon
- Black pepper – ¼ teaspoon
- Onion powder – ½ teaspoon
- Chopped parsley – 2 teaspoons
- Chopped dill – 1 tablespoon
- Unsweetened soy milk – ½ cup

Method of Preparation:

1. Whisk all of the ingredients, except the milk, together until well blended and add soy milk as desired.

Tip: You can swap mayonnaise with vegan sour cream for a tasty sauce.

Nutritional Information per serving:

- Calories: 93 Kcal
- Carbohydrates: 0 g
- Fat: 9 g
- Proteins: 0 g

Vegan Nacho Cheese

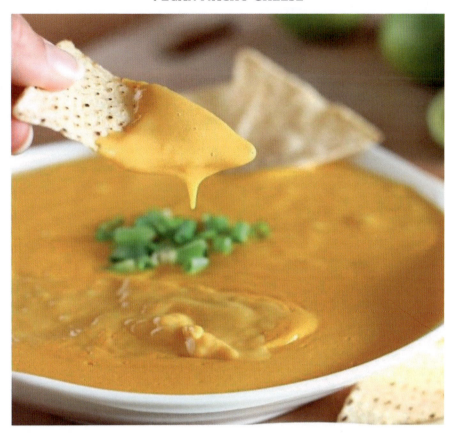

Preparation Time: 5 Minutes
Cooking Time: 15 Minutes
Servings: 6

Ingredients:

- Potatoes peeled– 2 cups (2 1/2 medium potatoes)
- Chopped carrots – 3/4 cup
- Nutritional yeast flakes – 1/2 cup
- Olive oil – 1/3 cup
- Lemon juice – 1 tablespoon
- Salt to taste
- Water – 1/3 cup

Method of Preparation:

1. Bring a pan of medium-large size of water to the boil.
2. Boil carrots and potatoes until tender then add to the blender and mash them.
3. Place all of the remaining ingredients into the blender and blend for 30 seconds or until completely smooth.
4. Serve the dip immediately with crackers, chips or toast. You can refrigerate the leftovers using an airtight container for 1 week.

Nutritional Information per serving:

- Calories: 28 K cal
- Carbohydrates: 3 g
- Fat: 1 g
- Proteins: 1 g

Ginger Cranberry Sauce

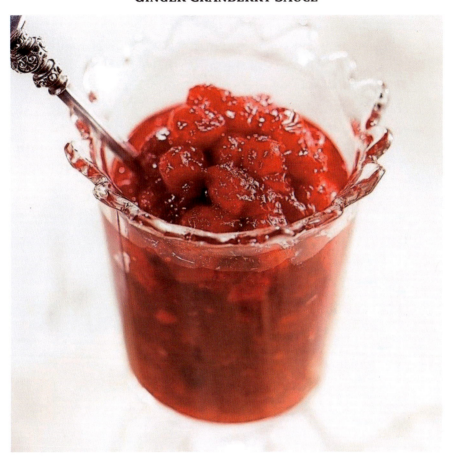

Preparation Time: 10 Minutes
Cooking Time: 5 Minutes
Servings: 8

Ingredients:

- Maple syrup – 1/2 cup
- Sugar – 1/3 cup
- Lime juice – 2 tablespoons
- Cranberries – 3 cups
- Fresh ginger, finely chopped – 1 teaspoon
- Water – ½ cup

Method of Preparation:

1. In a saucepan, you can stir together the maple syrup, lime juice, water and sugar and bring to a boil over medium heat. Keep stirring util the sugar dissolves. Reduce the heat and allow the mixture to simmer, uncovered, for about 3 minutes.
2. Add ginger and cranberries. Return to a boil and reduce the heat. Let it simmer for 5 minutes, uncovered, or until the berries have popped and the sauce begins to thicken. Keep stirring occasionally then remove from heat and allow to cool.

Tip: Instead of using sugar, you can also opt for sugar substitutes

Nutritional Information per serving:

- Calories: 83 Kcal
- Carbohydrates: 22 g
- Fat: 0 g
- Proteins:0 g

Vegan Green Chile Cilantro Sauce

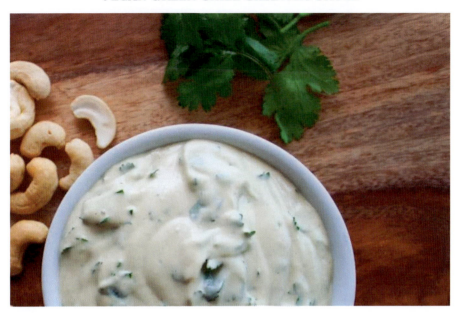

Preparation Time: 10 Minutes
Cooking Time: 0 Minutes
Servings: 4

Ingredients:

- Diced green chiles – 1 can (4 ounces)
- Raw unsalted cashews – 1 cup
- Hemp milk – ¼ cup
- Salt – ½ teaspoon
- Cilantro – 1 cup
- Jalapeño with seeds – 1, to taste

Method of Preparation:

1. In a blender process the green chiles, cashews, jalapeño and salt until smooth.
2. Add milk and blend again to combine, then pour the mixture into a bowl.
3. Chop cilantro and stir into the cashew and milk mixture.

4. Store in the refrigerator covered until you intend to serve.

Tip: Cashews are normally used as a non-dairy base.

Nutritional Information per serving:

- ➤ Calories: 93 Kcal
- ➤ Carbohydrates: 14 g
- ➤ Fat: 6g
- ➤ Proteins:2 g

TOMATO SAUCE

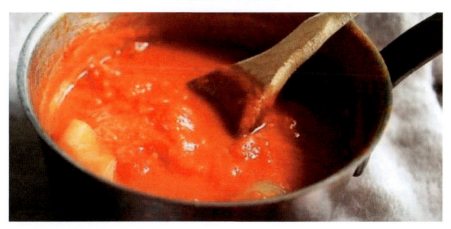

Preparation Time: 45 Minutes
Cooking Time: 5 Minutes
Servings: 4

Ingredients:

- Tomatoes – 2 cups (whole peeled tomatoes with juices)
- Unsalted Butter – 5 tablespoons
- Onion, chopped – 1 medium
- Salt to taste

Method of Preparation:

1. Combine the tomatoes and juices, onion, butter and salt in a saucepan.
2. Place your pan over medium heat and bring to a simmer. Cook for 45 minutes, stirring occasionally.
3. Discard the onions and taste for salt. Use as a sauce with pasta.
4. Serve and enjoy

Tip: You can add as many herbs as desired for additional flavor.

Nutritional Information per serving:

- Calories: 18 Kcal
- Carbohydrates: 3 g
- Fat: 0.2 g
- Proteins: 0.9 g

CHIPOTLE AIOLI

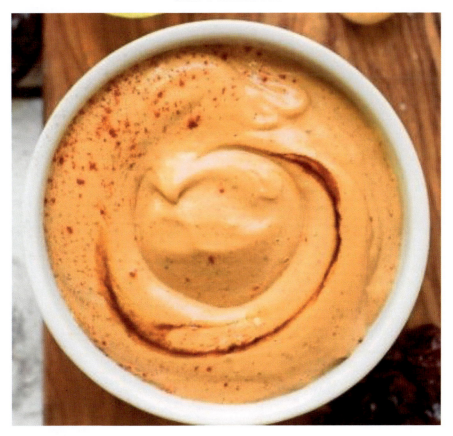

Preparation Time: 45 Minutes
Cooking Time: 15 Minutes
Servings: 8

Ingredients:

- Raw cashews – ¾ cup
- Unsweetened plain almond milk – ½ cup
- Lemon juice – 2 tablespoon
- Sea salt – ¼ teaspoon
- Whole chipotle peppers – 3
- Avocado oil, canola oil, grapeseed oil or any other natural oil – 1 teaspoon

- Smoked paprika – optional

Method of Preparation:

1. Cover the cashews with hot water in a bowl and let sit for an hour. Drain.
2. Add the soaked and drained cashews to a high-speed blender with the almond milk, maple syrup, pepper, sea salt, oil and lemon juice and blend until well mixed.
3. Taste and adjust as desired. Serve immediately or refrigerate. You can keep the leftovers, covered and refrigerated, for about 7 days.

Tip: Adjust the seasonings depending on the intensity of the taste you desire.

Nutritional Information per serving:

- Calories: 73 Kcal
- Carbohydrates: 6 g
- Fat: 5.2 g
- Proteins: 2 g

Romesco Sauce

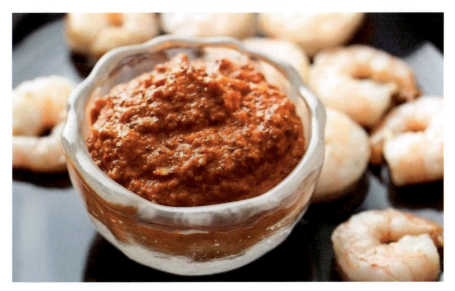

Preparation Time: 45 Minutes
Cooking Time: 15 Minutes
Servings: 8

Ingredients:

- Medium tomato - ½
- Peeled garlic cloves – 2 medium
- Crusty bread – 2 slices
- Red wine vinegar - 2 tablespoons
- Smoked paprika - 1/2 teaspoon
- Whole raw almonds – ¼ cup
- Roasted red peppers, drained – 1 cup
- Olive oil – ¼ cup
- Kosher salt – 1 teaspoon

Method of Preparation:

1. Preheated the oven to 450^0F and place the rack in the middle.

2. Arrange tomatoes, almonds, bread and garlic on a rimmed baking sheet and roast until the almonds and bread are toasted slightly.
3. Transfer all toasted ingredients to a food processor and pulse until coarsely chopped. Add roasted peppers, olive oil, vinegar, paprika and salt and pulse again until smooth and well combined.
4. Serve and enjoy or refrigerate.

Nutritional Information per serving:

- Calories: 301 Kcal
- Carbohydrates: 16 g
- Fat: 24 g
- Proteins: 5 g

Vegan Chocolate Sauce

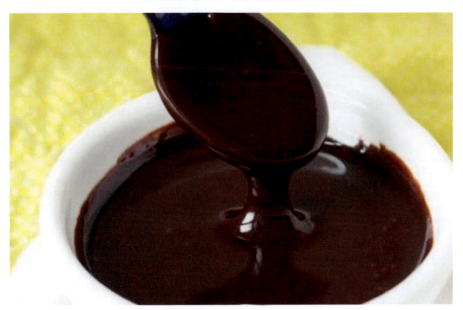

Preparation Time: 45 Minutes
Cooking Time: 15 Minutes
Servings: 8

Ingredients:

- Coconut milk – 14 ounces
- Cocoa powder – 1/3 cup
- Sugar – ½ cup
- Refined coconut oil – 2 tablespoons
- Vanilla extract – ½ teaspoon

Method of Preparation:

1. Whisk together the sugar, cocoa powder and coconut milk until well blended.
2. Pour the ready mixture into a saucepan and bring to a boil. Let simmer lightly , constantly stirring, for about 10 minutes.

3. Remove from the heat. Add the coconut oil and vanilla extract and stir until well blended.
4. Allow the sauce to cool and it will keep in an airtight container, refrigerated, for about one week.
5. Serve when desired and enjoy.

Tip: Can be used over vegan ice cream or as a dessert itself.

Nutritional Information per serving:

- Calories: 230 Kcal
- Carbohydrates: 1 2g
- Fat: 4 g
- Proteins: 2 g

Miso–Ginger Sauce

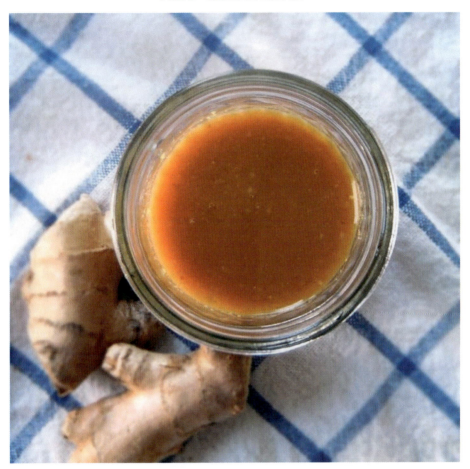

Preparation Time: 15 Minutes
Cooking Time: 10 Minutes
Servings: 2

Ingredients:

- Dark sesame oil – 1 tablespoon
- Thinly sliced large onion – 1
- Unbleached white flour – 1½ Cup
- Minced garlic clove – 2
- Grated fresh ginger – 1 tablespoon

- White Miso – 3 tablespoons
- Sesame seeds - 1 tablespoon
- Cayenne pepper – pinch
- Dried hot pepper flakes, optional

Method of Preparation:

1. First place a saucepan over medium heat and add the oil. Add the onion and sauté until translucent. Add garlic and continue to sauté until onion is lightly browned.
2. Sprinkle in the flour and stir until it dissolves, then stir in the ginger. Combine the miso with about ¾ cup of water and whisk in a bowl until well combined. Pour the miso slowly into the saucepan and allow to simmer for 4 minutes over low heat.
3. Add sesame seeds and cayenne. Adjust the consistency using water if the sauce is too thick. Remove from heat.
4. Serve immediately and enjoy.

Tip: You can toss it with cooked noodles or serve with some steamed broccoli.

Nutritional Information per serving:

- Calories: 182 Kcal
- Carbohydrates: 7 g
- Fat:3 g
- Proteins:2 g

7-Day Vegan Meal Plan

Sessions	Day 1	Day 2	Day 3	Day 4	Day 5	Day 5	Day 7
Breakfast	Chocolate Strawberry Oatmeal	Vegan Pancakes	Overnight Blueberry Oats	Vegan Keto Porridge	Pear and Walnut Oatmeal	Easy Vegan Oatmeal	Vegan Quinoa Porridge
Lunch	Kale & sweet potato salad	Spinach chickpeas	Spinach pan casserole	Broccoli Salad with Peanut	Kale & sweet potato salad	Tofu Scramble	Grilled Eggplant
Snack	Chocolate chunk cookies	Blueberry quinoa bran muffins	Energy balls	Apple sweet potato hash	Pumpkin Biscuit	Chocolate chunk cookies	Chocolate chunk cookies
Dinner	Broccoli Salad with Peanut	Spanakopita mashed potatoes	Coconut Curry	Roasted pumpkin and chickpea salad	Tomato and garlic butter bean	Healthy Oatmeal	Vegan Banana Bread
Dessert	Golden Milk Smoothie	Peanut butter oatmeal	Coconut Ice cream	Savory Oatmeal	Strawberry chickpea pudding	Peanut butter oatmeal	Carrot cake oatmeal

CONCLUSION

Congratulations! And thank you for taking the time to read this book. **Rainbow Vegan Cookbook** has covered in detail what a vegan diet entails, and how you can successfully transition to a vegan lifestyle. The book is fully packed with healthy and nutritious recipes that can help you succeed in adopting a vegan lifestyle.

Now that you have the right information and how you can get started, go ahead and implement the information you have read.

I do have a small request: would you kindly take the time to leave a review of this book!

Congratulations! All the best in following a vegan lifestyle!

Printed by Amazon Italia Logistica S.r.l.
Torrazza Piemonte (TO), Italy